T0354989

YOUR LEGS

OR

YOUR LIFE?

OTHER BOOKS BY JIM MEEHAN

Hearts Have Reasons
(UK Outword Trust 1995; USA Thomas Moore 2000)

Reasons Have Hearts Too
(UK Outword Trust 1997; USA Thomas Moore 2000)

Sugar Free Sweet Talk
(USA Talent Plus 2009)

Hallways to Success and Significance
(USA Talent Plus 2013)

I Mean You No Harm; I Seek Your Greatest Good – Reflections on Trust
(USA I Universe 2015)

Armless Hugs
(USA I Universe 2020)

YOUR LEGS OR YOUR LIFE?

JIM MEEHAN

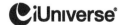

YOUR LEGS OR YOUR LIFE?

iUniverse books may be ordered through booksellers or by contacting:

iUniverse
1663 Liberty Drive
Bloomington, IN 47403
www.iuniverse.com
844-349-9409

ISBN: 978-1-6632-6372-8 (sc)
ISBN: 978-1-6632-6373-5 (e)

Library of Congress Control Number: 2024911573

Print information available on the last page.

iUniverse rev. date: 12/19/2024

This book is dedicated to all amputees
and the people who care for them.

All proceeds from sales will be donated to the
United Kingdom Limbless Association
whose vision is that 'no amputee need cope alone.'

CONTENTS

LIST OF ILLUSTRATIONS

Photos

Figures

When the surgeons cut off my legs beneath my knees,
They cut off a much deeper part of me.
Now, in many things, I am less independent and free.
A partial burden for others to carry.

Yes, I'm grateful to be alive and no longer in severe pain,
And having the potential to walk again,
Albeit with the aid of crutches or a mobility frame,
And drive a car or travel by train or plane.

But to heal fully what can I say?
Well, I need to hope more and try not to dismay.
Adopt a more positive approach day by day.
And deepen my human relationships in every way.

Jim Meehan
August 2023

INTRODUCTION

On March 11th 2022, six months before my 80th birthday, I had my left leg amputated below the knee. Prior to this surgery I recall lying in my hospital bed, surrounded by a team of vascular consultants who were explaining my options which were, more or less, boiled down to a choice I had to make. "It's your leg or your life?"

On April 13th 2023, seven months after my 80th birthday, I had my right leg amputated below the knee. Prior to this surgery I recall being informed by Mrs. Rachel Sam, senior vascular consultant of several West Midlands University Hospitals, that my gangrene infested right foot was beyond repair and asking my permission to arrange the planned amputation of my right leg below the knee.

All my family, friends, neighbours, many former work colleagues and clients have been somewhat dumbfounded by the deterioration of my health over the last four and a half years. They thought, like I did, that I was quite fit and was someone who would have a long and healthy aerobic life.

Over this period of time, I have had to deal with some excruciating physical and nervous pain and had to make major adjustments to my life expectations. On a couple of occasions,

I felt close to death's door. In addition, I have had plenty of time to reflect on my health and fitness story and the steps I have taken to aid my recovery.

All of which made me think that it could be of some benefit to share with others the lessons I have learned from this experience and at the same time reinforce key aspects of my psychological approach to life.

So, I hope you enjoy following my health and fitness journey, learning about my coping strategies and insights and that they will enable you, to some extent, to live a fuller, healthier and happier life.

Jim Meehan
May 2024

PART ONE

MY HEALTH AND
FITNESS STORY

"Love set you going like a fat gold watch.
The midwife slapped your footsoles,
and your bald cry
Took its place among the elements."

Sylvia Plath
Morning Song 1961.

Love set me going, as Sylvia Plath poetically put it, during the Christmas season of 1941. Nine months later my first cry, which by all family accounts was 'bold' not 'bald', was heard on 20th September in Walton Park Hospital, 107 Rice Lane, Liverpool, England. It could be said that it was my first experience of being in hospital, albeit not one committed to conscious memory.

It was in the middle of World War II. A time of food rationing and the breaking up of families as mothers and children were sent to safe places outside the line of fire. My mother, Margaret, had to travel to Birkdale, the home of one of the UK's Open Golf Championship Courses near to the seaside resort of Southport, thirty miles northwest of Liverpool, in May 1941. There she gave birth to my elder brother, John. It was a time for air-raid sirens, bombs, shelters and gas masks (which, in 1945, I thought were toys). But it was also a time of courage, determination and British 'bulldog-grit.'

When my birth was registered, the certificate confirmed that my father, John, had been conscripted as a private in the Army and was attached to a local aircraft manufacturing factory as a timekeeper. My father, mother and my elder brother, John, lived in a family commune, comprising six adults and two children, at my paternal grandfather's house in 51 Ampthill Road, in the well-appointed suburb of Aigburth, Liverpool.

Following the transfer of my father from Liverpool, my mother took my brother and me to stay in Seaforth, a dockland suburb where she was born in 1917 during the first World War. My mother was stone deaf in her right ear and nervously deaf in her left ear, which meant that she could not hear people she did not know well. She wanted to be closer to her mother and father, her seven siblings and their families and to her former friends. We lived with her maternal Aunt Helen, a spinster, in a 'two-up and two-down' property with one outside toilet at 12 Beaumaris Street.

It was the only time I can remember as a child being under nourished. One morning I asked my aunt what was for breakfast and she quipped "Three jumps at the pantry door," which was her way of saying the pantry was bare. Often, I would faint at school until I was given the daily milk allowance. Money was frequently in short supply because we were dependent on funds sent by my father, which were often delayed in the mail.

My father, who could speak French, was sent to Mechelen in Belgium to serve with some Canadian troops. This meant that he was late in being demobilized. Unfortunately, when he returned home there was a shortage of suitable jobs available for him in Liverpool. Nevertheless, he immediately arranged for our family to return to his father's house in 51 Ampthill Road, Aigburth.

The first time I used the United Kingdom's National

Health Service (NHS) was during our time in Aigburth. I was nearly six years old when Aneurin Bevan set up the NHS on 5th July 1948. One Saturday morning, I was asked to go to the butchers in Aigburth Vale to collect some pork sausages and a joint of meat. On the way I played a game which involved rolling my school cap into a rugby ball which I tossed high into the air and which I caught before it hit the ground.

Aigburth Vale was a main road adjoining Ampthill Road, running below an embankment along which electric trams travelled to and from the city-centre and the suburbs of Dingle, Aigburth, Garston and Speke. As I was crossing the tramlines I tossed my cap high in the air and it perched on top of a pole supporting the overhead electric wires. Next, I successfully shimmied up the pole and as I was reaching for my cap a tram passed by and I felt a jolt and passed out. I woke up three days later, after being in a coma, in the Royal Liverpool Children's Hospital, asking for pork sausages and a joint of meat.

I was told that I had fallen almost fifteen feet from the pole onto the embankment and then rolled over and fell onto the roof of the toilets in Aigburth Vale below and finally fell on to the road in front of the butchers in a state of unconsciousness. An ambulance was called and rushed me to hospital. Fortunately, no bones were broken but the doctors kept me in hospital for a week or so after coming out of the coma, for further observation.

I do not recall experiencing any severe pain while in hospital but I remember on one night there was a great commotion in the ward. A patient who was heavily bandaged and fitted with several drips and surrounded by many doctors and nurses was wheeled into the bay next to mine. He was being carefully monitored. Later I learned that it was a boy who had been stealing lead from the roof of the Liverpool Anglian Cathedral and had fallen from a great height. Unfortunately, he died the next day. Somewhat scared, I thanked my lucky stars that my team of doctors and nurses had been able to help me regain consciousness and keep from further harm.

I was also told that a boy knocked on the door of our house shortly after the fall and when my mother opened the door, he shouted, "There's something wrong with your Jimmy's head" and my mother replied "I know," and shut the door. My mother probably did not hear or understand exactly what the boy had said. However, the story spread like wildfire!

As a small boy I was always climbing, starting with what appeared to me, at the time, to be steep cliffs lining the cast iron or "cassie" shore on the banks of the River Mersey, near to Aigburth. The climbing was quite dangerous but extremely exhillerating. Other solo pursuits I enjoyed were climbing to the tops of trees in Sefton Park, Aigburth and clambering over the ruins of Sefton Park's Victorian Palm House which was in a state of disrepair following a nearby bomb-blast in 1941 which had dislodged most of its glass, leaving many empty frames. I had a head for heights and I loved jumping off the top diving board at Garston's public swimming baths.

Soon after I had been fully discharged from hospital my father arranged for our family to move to England's second largest city Birmingham, where he got a job as a bus conductor. We lived in a pleasant suburb called Acocks Green where my father rented a property on Yardley Road whose back garden backed onto a canal.

While I never became a distinguished performer, record breaker or team captain I was always an enthusiastic and competitive participant in sports. I represented my primary schools at football, cricket and athletics and became a successful junior high board diver. Likewise, when I went to Saint Philip's Secondary Grammar School, in the wealthy suburb of Edgbaston, Birmingham I represented my House, at football, swimming and cricket. I recall with pride at the age of seventeen achieving tenth place out of a field of over 150, sixteen-to-eighteen-year-old male participants, in an annual seven and a half-mile cross-country race. Often, as a teenager, I would borrow my elder brother's bicycle and cycle to local tourist centres like Coventry City, Stratford - Upon - Avon and Warwick. At college I was in the football team and enjoyed solo cross country running and cycling. After leaving college on 23rd February 1965, my elder brother John and I joined a local Sunday football team, Hurst Rangers, for a couple of seasons.

Around this time my other brother, Stephen, who is eight years younger than me, decided he would like to join me on a challenging cycling holiday, namely, to ride the 195-mile world famous, scenic Antrim Coast Road in Northern Ireland which started in Belfast and finished in Londonderry.

To limber up for the challenge we rode 120 miles to Liverpool and then boarded a boat which sailed to Douglas on the Isle of Man, in the Irish Sea. There we cycled around the famous 38-mile Touring Trophy (TT) Motor-bike circuit and gained experience of riding up and down steep mountain trails. We also got used to sleeping in youth hostels. When feeling fighting-fit we boarded a boat which sailed to Belfast in Northern Ireland. This was followed by a few days of restful sight-seeing before we took on our challenge.

The vistas were majestic, especially the number one highlight, The Giant's Causeway, declared a World Heritage Site in 1986 by UNESCO. The views from the many bridges we crossed on our way to Londonderry were spectacular too. However, the weather was very wet and blustery. We certainly needed our shower capes and sou'westers. All in all, it was well worth the tremendous effort.

Mission accomplished, we then crossed the border into Donegal in Eire just to put our feet outside of Great Britain, before heading Southeast to Ballymena where we put our bikes on a train. We disembarked at the port of Larne on the bank of the North Sea. From there we boarded a ferry to Stranraer on the West coast of Scotland. Finally, we put our bikes on another train and had a restful journey back to Birmingham City.

During the nineteen eighties I joined a local mountain walking club made up of work colleagues from Rover Cars Manufacturing Company, where I then worked, and a few nearby friends. Often it involved weekend camping trips. We walked up the highest peaks in the British Isles, namely, Scafell Pike (England 3,209 ft.) Snowden (Wales 3,560 ft.) Ben Nevis (Scotland 4,143 ft.) and Carrauntoohil (Eire 3,407 ft.). We also scaled many peaks in the southeast of France, in central Germany, in the Austrian and Italian Alps, and in the

Spanish Pyrenees. In 1991, after I moved to the United States to become the Director of Psychological Services for a start-up International Human Resources Consultancy, Talent Plus, I was able to walk in the Rockies and reached the summit of Grays Peak (14,278 ft.) on the International Divide in the state of Colorado. In addition, I had the pleasure of walking many ski slopes and mountain peaks in the west of Canada, north of Vancouver and also in the Blue Mountains in the east of Canada, not far from the Niagara Falls.

On my health journey I have had a few set-backs. For instance, on 24th March 1996, my wife's fifty third birthday, when I was diagnosed as having late onset Type II diabetes. Initially, I thought I was suffering from jet-lag as I had been working in ski resorts across Canada and in many hotels throughout the USA, including the islands of Hawaii. In addition, I was also responsible for liaising with many pub managers throughout the United Kingdom.

My UK doctor told me that I was burning the candle at both ends, jet-setting and at times working eighteen-hour days writing psychological portraits of clients. He also stressed the need for me to adopt a better work-life balance and avoid the risk of a total burn-out. He urged me to eat fewer carbohydrates and exercise more. It was at this time that I decided to control my blood glucose levels by diet and increase my physical exercise regimen. Interestingly, nobody could give me the precise cause of my diabetes as there was no family history of the disease. I was even told that many war-time babies, like me, who were on food rations and at times undernourished, developed Type II diabetes later in life.

In the United States I became a member of the Juvenile Diabetes Research Foundation (JDRF) and helped to plan and participate in walks to raise money for a cure for people with Type I diabetes, who required insulin to live.

Another set-back occurred on 12th January 2002 when I slipped on ice as I was walking to the gym early in the morning. I went head over heels and on landing I heard a crack in my left foot and when pushing up I heard another crack in the same foot. I assumed that something had popped out and then popped back in place. Next, I climbed seventeen steps, entered my apartment and had a shower. On my way to work my ankle swelled into a balloon as I was driving, so I pulled in to the local accident and emergency department at Bryan Hospital, Lincoln, Nebraska. I informed the main receptionist that I thought I had sprained my left ankle. She told me to go to the podiatry section which was 250 yards away. On arrival, a nurse told me to sit in the waiting room and let me know that a podiatrist would examine me in due course. After fifteen minutes or so a young man arrived and took off my shoe. Startled, he said "I hope you have not walked on this as your foot has been completely severed from your ankle." That night under general anaesthetic, a surgeon attached a titanium plate to the side of my left calf and ankle and using titanium screws fixed my foot to the plate.

In early 2004 Talent Plus received an award for the funds the company had raised for JDRF walks. At that event the chairperson asked for volunteers to cycle through Death Valley Desert in California to raise funds for research into Type I diabetes. I threw my hat in the ring, unaware of what was fully involved and was joined shortly after by three work colleagues from Talent Plus. We began training in March 2004 for the race which was set to take place in October 2004. All the riders were allocated Youth Ambassadors whose role was to support their riders in raising funds. My Youth Ambassador was a beautiful ten-year-old girl, Stacie Post, who had been diagnosed with Type I diabetes in her early childhood. I had her photo attached to my handlebars to inspire me over the gruelling seven-month training period and the actual ride. After two months of training one of our male riders had to drop out as he had been diagnosed with prostate cancer.

Ten days before the race I was involved in a road accident. I was riding on a cycle track during training. I came to a road junction where I thought I had right of way. I saw a special utility vehicle (SUV), come to the junction and stop. Accordingly, I continued but the driver suddenly accelerated and hit me full on. I had no time to detach myself from my bike and, it and I, became trapped under the vehicle. The driver called an ambulance and the paramedics managed to extricate me from my bike and drag me onto the sidewalk. I was bleeding profusely from my head and my cycle-helmet was cracked in two places. They took me and my bike to Saint Elizabeth's, the local hospital and after several x-rays the doctors told me there were no broken bones but my bike was a total write off.

Fortunately, I contacted the rider with prostate cancer, who had dropped out of our team and from the funds I eventually received as a result of a successful insurance claim, bought his road bike so that I could still participate in the ride. On

23rd October 2004 three of us from Talent Plus completed the 105-mile course through the desert, involving a descent to 282 feet below sea level and also included a seven mile one-in-five gradient mountain climb. The average temperature was close to 100 degrees Fahrenheit and we often had to ride into 50 mile per hour headwinds. We raised over $10,000 for JDRF. I found out later that my ambassador, Stacie got up early on that day hoping to cheer the riders on.

My confidence to participate in endurance sports grew and soon I began training to run a full-marathon. However, after I ran fourteen miles my hamstring muscles pulled. A leading physiotherapist, who trained the Lincoln girl's-college basketball team, told me I would not be able to run a full marathon because the metal in my left foot and ankle caused my hamstrings to pull after running fourteen miles. Accordingly, he tried to restrict me to a half-marathon run only. However, I decided to get fitted with a double pair of Spandex ski-tights to keep my hamstrings tightly attached to my thigh bones and had expensive orthotics made in Sioux City to line my trainers and thereby provide more foot support. In addition, I read about the need to avoid "hitting the wall," which resulted in many runners losing strength and eventually failing to complete the run. The experts recommended running 400 miles over 16 to 18 weeks before the race in which to build up sufficient glycogen. They pointed out that a reasonably healthy person could run 20 miles based on their normal resources but needed enough glycogen to complete the last 6 miles. Eventually, I joined several colleagues at Talent

Plus and completed my first full-marathon run at Lincoln, Nebraska in May 2008 at the age of sixty-five.

Then I began running and cycling daily for the next few years and in May 2010 completed the Lincoln Marathon again and in October 2012 for my 70th birthday I finished the Chicago Marathon but had to run with cotton buds in my nose to stop bleeding that had started a week before the run.

After resigning from Talent Plus on 30th April 2015 Maureen and I returned to the United Kingdom so we could be closer to our daughter, Larissa and our grandson, Amir, who had been born on 8th January 2015. I continued to work, but this time as a freelance positive British Chartered Psychologist, keynote speaker, author and published poet.

It wasn't long before I volunteered to raise funds to support Diabetes UK by running the Great North Run, the world's largest half-marathon in terms of participants. In October 2016, at the age of seventy-four, I successfully completed the run.

For the next few years daily running or cycling were the main ingredients of my physical fitness regimen. The mountain walkers had renamed their club to become the SWALLOWS, meaning, Short Walks and Long Lunches on Wednesdays!

In March 2018, for my wife's 75th birthday, we travelled to South America where we spent time initially exploring the capital of Argentina, Buenos Aries, and visiting Uruguay. We then flew north to Brazil and spent time walking to the Iguazu Water Falls. At a length of 2.8 kilometres, they are the world's biggest falls, bordering both Argentina and Brazil. During our stay in South America, I noticed that when we walked over seven miles my feet began to hurt and I felt the need to buy some new trainers but decided to wait until we returned to England.

On our return, my physiotherapist made some adjustments to my orthotics which provided adequate short-term pain relief. He felt that over the previous decade I had lost a lot of fat from the soles of my feet and that I was walking virtually on bone.

In 2019 Maureen and I were invited by Talent Plus to attend the Nebraska State Capital where the State Governor celebrated the life and work of Dr. William E. Hall, my psychological mentor, for his contribution to society and nominated his birthday, 19th August that year to his memory.

While in Lincoln we spoke with a friend who was recovering from major heart by-pass surgery. He told us that he was given a full bill of health by a local physician when he had his annual health check. However, another friend was given the same result by the same physician the previous year, but two weeks later died from a massive heart attack. Accordingly, our friend decided to take a Computer Tomography Coronary Calcium Screening Test which was on offer at the local hospital. He discovered that his arteries were highly calcified and he was admitted the next day for major heart surgery. He urged me to undergo the same procedure before I left Lincoln. I took his advice and the day before we returned to England I was duly screened.

The results were received a week or so later and indicated that I needed further assessment by a cardiologist, including stress testing. In December 2019 I was diagnosed with asymptomatic intermittent atrial fibrillation, an irregular heart-beat, which required anti-coagulant medication. A follow-up ultrasound scan of my heart, however, revealed that my heart was normal and that no further action was required on that front.

Following this my running, walking and cycling performances became erratic and the soles of my feet began to hurt so much that I could no longer run and walked in pain. My physiotherapist agreed to see me in the first week of January 2021 to examine my trainers, mountain boots, cycling shoes, dress shoes and slippers all of which needed the same orthotics to avoid irregular rubbing.

Then came a major set-back. On the 31st December 2020 after having a shower, following a five-mile run, I stubbed the second toe of my left foot against a dress shoe. It was very painful. The toe became inflamed and I managed to get an appointment with my podiatrist at the beginning of the New Year. She said that she thought the toenail was intact but that I needed to attend my diabetic review on 21st January 2021 in case antibiotics were required. The nurse at the diabetic clinic thought I had cellulitis and arranged for the doctor on duty to prescribe suitable antibiotics.

However, the antibiotics made no difference. My nail dropped off and revealed an ulcer so I was referred to the local hospital in Solihull where different and more powerful antibiotics were tried. When they failed, I was sent to see the senior vascular consultant of the Heartlands Regional Hospital, Mrs. Rachel Sam, who immediately arranged an ultrasound of my left leg. This showed that the blood flow in my groin was strong but was very weak in my calf and extremely weak in my foot. She next arranged for me to have an angiogram of the arteries in my left leg. This procedure involved a Radiologist conducting a special x-ray of blood vessels. Normally, blood vessels do not show up on ordinary x- rays. However, by injecting a special dye, called a contrast medium, into an artery through a plastic tube called a catheter, and taking x-rays afterwards, detailed images of arteries and veins can be produced.

On the 4th March 2021 I had the angiogram and a clot was discovered and successfully unblocked by a medical procedure known as an angioplasty which was given under local anaesthetic. However, in the longer term the nail refused to heal and gangrene set in. As I could no longer perform aerobic exercise, I was put on medications to control my blood glucose and cholesterol levels.

In November 2021 my right big toenail turned dark; this time without me having stubbed an object. An examination revealed that that there was an ulcer beneath the toenail which needed to be treated. I underwent another angiogram which again found that I had a clot in my right calf, which was successfully unblocked by another angioplasty. However, in the longer term the procedure failed to heal the big toenail and gangrene set in. So, now I had both feet with toes affected by gangrene.

At the beginning of March 2022, I began to sweat at night because of the severe pain and became so disoriented that I fell out of bed which made the gangrene on my left foot weep. I was rushed into the Regional NHS Hospital with symptoms of sepsis and ended up, as previously stated, having my left leg amputated below the knee on 11th March 2022.

Two months later I attended the West Midlands Amputee Rehabilitation Centre in Selly Oak, Birmingham to be assessed for a prosthetic leg to enable me to walk. However, because my right foot was not healing sufficiently the team decided to proceed with a prosthetic leg for transfer purposes only and not for walking. With the help of a wooden banana- shaped board I could get in and out of bed or in and out of the car.

In October 2022 I had the top of my right big toenail amputated under local anaesthetic and also had an angiogram and angioplasty but they failed to stop the deterioration of the wound and gangrene spread to three other toes on the foot. Despite a lot of debridement, involving the removal of dead, damaged or infected tissue to improve the healing potential of the remaining tissue, it became impossible to avoid the amputation of my right leg below the knee on the 13th April 2023.

I then received another appointment to attend the West Midlands Amputee Rehabilitation Centre in Selly Oak, Birmingham on 28th June 2023 for them to assess if I would be a suitable client for a second prosthetic leg, this time for the primary purpose of walking. In the meanwhile, I had a series of strenuous exercises to carry out to build up my muscles and increase my body's flexibility. On my 81st birthday, 20th September 2023 using a prosthetic leg on my left stump and aided by an air bag in a metal frame on my right stump (see Photo.1) I was able to stand and walk with the aid of parallel bars. Fortunately, the team agreed to proceed with the manufacture of a prosthetic leg for my right stump to enable me to walk on two artificial legs.

On 22nd December 2023 I was fitted with a prosthetic for my right stump and was able to walk several laps with the aid of parallel bars (see Photo.2) and also walked several metres along the corridors with the aid of a Zimmer frame (see Photo.3).

Shortly after, while I was sitting and reflecting in my wheelchair, on New Year's Day 2024, it seemed to me that as a child and school-boy I was reasonably active and keen to pursue individual events and engage in team sports too. At college I was more of an academic than a sportsman but realized that a healthy mind required a healthy body. Once I started my working career, acquiring the highest possible professional qualifications was my main priority during the sixties and seventies along with finding a life partner and starting a family. In the nineteen eighties mountain walking kept me fit during my forties. However, the biggest wake-up call as far as my health and fitness journey was concerned was being diagnosed with Type II diabetes in 1996 at the age of fifty-three. I was told at the time that there was no cure for Type II diabetes. This is no longer the case, as the condition has been reversed for many people.

"A persistent plodder," aptly described my athletic performance, particularly in the years prior to my amputations. Immediately after the amputations I found it difficult to accept fully that I will have to spend the rest of my life without any legs and all that implies. How I missed not being able to play football and tennis and going on holidays with my grandson, Amir, who was 9 years old on the 8th January 2024.

With hindsight, I think my approach to my health was possibly too narrow. While I thought my major health issue was being diagnosed with Type II diabetes which I focused upon by checking my blood glucose levels daily and maintaining them by exercising and controlling my carbohydrate intake, unfortunately, I had paid insufficient focus on my blood circulation, until it was too late. It was a lack of adequate blood flow that was the critical factor that prevented my infected feet from healing. It seems to me now that I needed to have paid more attention to my blood flow, maybe as soon as I was diagnosed with Type II diabetes in March 1996.

Certainly, I am taking a more broad-brush approach to my present and future health and fitness journey rather than compartmentalizing my focus and I would recommend my readers to adopt a holistic approach to their health and fitness journeys too.

We need to recognize that there are many hidden factors, such as our genetic make-up, that contribute to the deterioration of our well-being that are out of our control, but which we, nevertheless need to accept and respond to as best we can and not judge ourselves and others too harshly. In other words, we have to accept the vulnerability of being human beings. We all have our individual differences. No one is perfect. We all have our strengths and weaknesses. We all make mistakes.

By a strange coincidence on Friday 5th January 2024 Oscar Pistorius the famous athletic double leg amputee from South

Africa was being released from prison in Pretoria on parole, after serving eight and a half years in jail, by all accounts, as an ideal prisoner. Oscar, who was born on 28th November 1986 with congenital deformities of his ankles and feet, had his legs amputated just below the knees when he was only 11 months old. The story of how he rose from there to Paralympic glory and then take part in the Olympic Games in London in 2012 is one of the most amazing and inspirational stories I have come across. His motto is very positive- "You're not disabled by the disabilities you have; you are able by the abilities you have."

At the age of 26 his life was changed forever when he killed his beautiful 29-year-old girlfriend, Reeva Steenkamp, a model and trained lawyer, on Valentine's Day 2013, which he has always maintained was accidental and unintentional. John Carlin who followed in detail the legal proceedings and who had a three-hour interview with Oscar, during a mid-trial break, thinks that at the heart of the crime lies a mystery that may never be resolved. In an article Carlin wrote in the Sunday times on 31st December 2023, he concludes, "whatever exactly happened that Valentine's night, I think he has suffered enough now and deserves some peace."

In contrast to Oscar and Reeva, I did not become a double amputee until I was 80 years old and without my wife, Maureen, being by my side I would surely would have died by now. She has been an unsung hero. For a period of 100 days while our bathroom was being converted into a wet-room she had to give me a daily body-wash and even today helps me to take a daily shower. She detects and treats bed sores on my body and blisters on my stumps. She has had to manage my various medicines, which at peak pain and infestation times, mounted to over 20 pills to be taken over a 24-hour period; some to be taken an hour before meals, some during meals and some two hours after meals and some during the night. She cooks all my meals in strict accordance with my diabetic diet. In addition, she has been my cheerful chauffeur, having to put up with a neurotic front seat driver in the process! Without her help I am unable to travel by car as she has to dismantle my wheelchair by removing the wheels and folding it up before storing it in the back of the car. Moreover, she ensures that my many appointments are met on time, whether it is with my general practitioner for blood tests and injections, with various hospital professionals, or for regular dental, eye, hairdressing appointments and social events. Most important of all, is her constant companionship, friendship and loving kindness.

Not to forget that I am also very fortunate to have the care and attention of my daughter, Larissa who provides me with holistic therapies, particularly when it comes to relieving joint and muscle pain by way of massage therapy. She too acts as a chauffeur at times.

On the general question of human vulnerability, I recall in 1996 writing a few verses to Maureen which were eventually shaped into a poem called "Enough is Enough."

You have always been my enough,
I never expected you to be perfect.
People are not made of such stuff,
In function or form free of any defect.

Thank you for accepting me as your enough,

For allowing me sometimes to get it wrong.
For selectively calling my bluff,
Whenever my dances did not match my songs.

Today I think I would write, "You have always been much more than my enough."

These verses are an apt segue into the next chapter about embracing the healing power of good human relationships.

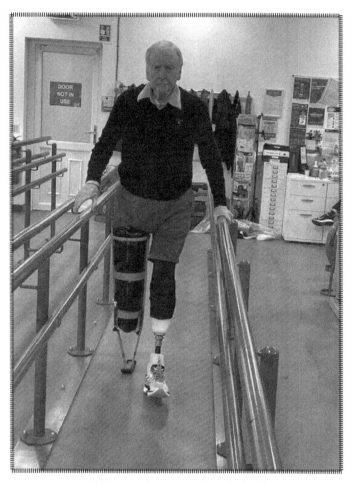

Photo 1. Walking with a prosthetic leg and air bag with the aid of parallel bars, September 2023.

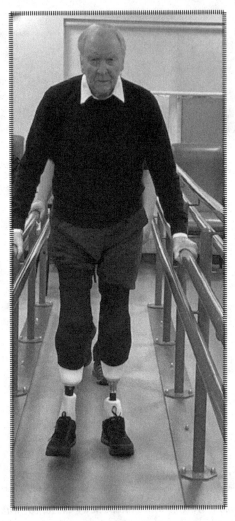

Photo 2. Walking with two prosthetic legs with the
aid of parallel bars, December 2023.

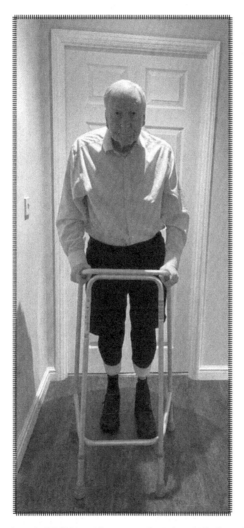

Photo 3. Walking with two prosthetic legs with the aid of a Zimmer frame, December 2023.

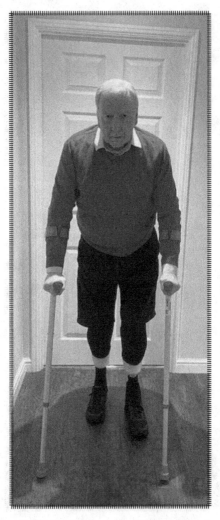

Photo 4. Walking with two prosthetic legs with the aid of two arm-length crutches, May 2024.

PART TWO

STEPS TAKEN TO AID MY ONGOING RECOVERY

STEP ONE

EMBRACING THE HEALING POWER OF GOOD HUMAN RELATIONSHIPS

"The major difficulty of relationships today
is that they are un-reflected actions."
Dr William E. Hall 1908-1998

Most of us, we can safely assume, came into this world as a result of a loving sexual relationship and that we survive and develop to our full human potential by the help we receive from other people. Human beings are essentially a social and inter-dependent species. Dr. Hall, my psychological mentor, never took human relationships for granted but reflected on key relationships daily and considered carefully what action he needed to take in the presence of others - acquaintances and strangers alike. He encouraged everybody else to do likewise. For him ignorance was never bliss when it came to good relationships. Although he was a pioneer positive psychologist, the father of strength psychology and success psychology he was above all a prominent good human relationship psychologist. He focused on identifying each person's potential but realized that just because a person has potential does not mean that he or she will activate that potential. For him, the best way to activate a person's potential is to have a good relationship with them or help them to have a good relationship with someone trustworthy and with high potential too. He was obsessed with measuring human personalities and distinguishing between top and average performers and between trustworthy and untrustworthy ones. For his 89th birthday I wrote a poem for him which tried to capture his vision, which I called "Picture a World".

Picture a world where each person was fully
employed
In doing good things they were good at,
intended and passionately enjoyed!
A place where due recognition was given and
people became the best that they can,
Significance shining in the eyes of every child,
woman and man.

Picture a world where each person was fully
engaged,
In positively making a difference, whatever
their strengths, race, religion or age.
A place where trusting relationships were
valued above all.
Welcome to the dreamland of a certain Doctor
William E. Hall.

Much scientific evidence shows that without good
relationships babies die or their growth is severely stunted.
For instance, there is the famous account of an experiment
allegedly carried out by Emperor Frederick II Hohenstaufen
(1194 – 1250) which was recorded by the monk Salimbene di
Adaerick in his *Chronicles*. He reported that Frederick ordered
"foster mothers and nurses to suckle, bathe, and wash the
newly born children but in no way to prattle or speak with
them so he could have learnt whether they would speak the
Hebrew language or Greek or Latin or Arabic, or perchance
the tongue of their parents of whom they were born. But he
laboured in vain, for the children could not live without the

clapping of hands and gestures and gladness of countenance and blandishments." Although Frederick was attempting to discover the original human language, what he actually discovered was that children who were deprived of good human interactions failed to survive.

More recently in Romania during the 1960s the Communist government outlawed contraception and abortion. The president, Nicolae Ceauşescu, for economic reasons, wanted to increase the population of Romania and become a world power. However, over 170,000 babies were sent to orphanages as their parents could not afford to raise them. When the president was overthrown in 1989 the world was shocked by the way most of the orphans were mistreated, ignored and neglected and whose growth had been severely stunted. As a result of this social deprivation the orphans grew up intellectually impaired, their brains and bodies were underdeveloped increasing their risks of serious health problems. Children deprived of love find it hard to thrive in the world. If children's interactions instill in them a feeling of being unwanted or unworthy of love it is not possible for them to see themselves as anything other than worthless and behave in ways to support that view.

Humans have a nature that requires nurture. It matters how we treat our children, and it matters more than we knew a few decades ago. It is up to all of us to create a social world which can help the little brains of our youngsters to grow healthy and whole.

The modern theoretical physicist Carlo Rovelli in his brilliant bestselling book *The Order of Time, (2019)* when talking about human self-identity stresses the importance of other human beings in the process and states,

"We have shaped an idea of a 'human being' by interacting with others like ourselves......I believe that our notion of self stems from this, not from introspection. When we think of ourselves as persons, I believe that we are applying to ourselves the mental circuits that we have developed to engage with our companions ...... The first image I have of myself as a child is the child my mother sees. We are for ourselves in large measure what we see and have seen of ourselves reflected back to us by our friends, our lovers and our enemies. I have never been convinced by the idea, attributed to Descartes, that the primary aspect of our experience is awareness of thinking, and therefore of existing....... The experience of oneself as a subject is not a primary experience: it is a complex cultural deduction, made on the basis of many other thoughts. My primary experience.....is to see the world around me, not myself. I believe we each have a concept of 'myself' only because at a certain point we learn to project on to ourselves the idea of being human as an additional feature that evolution has led us to develop during the course of millennia in order to engage with other members of our group: we are a reflection of the idea of ourselves that we receive back from our kind."

I am sure that Carlo would agree with the inscription that the ancient Greeks posted on the sun god, Apollo's temple in Delphi- *KNOW THYSELF* but would add *BY INTERRACTING WITH OTHERS*.

I recall attending a Talent Plus annual conference in Lincoln Nebraska in July 2007 where the key speaker, Dr. Mike

Neale, started by asking attendees to reflect on a statement attributed to the American sociologist Charles Horton Cooley (1864-1929) which goes as follows, "I am not who I think I am. I am not who you I think I am. I am who I think you think I am," which elegantly tries to encapsulate the role that others play in the formation of a person's self-concept and which tries to shed some light on the meaning of the expressions, "people are known by the company they keep," and "companies are known by the people they keep."

As was said earlier, we can safely assume that most people come into the world as a result of a loving sexual relationship and that we don't grow without nurturing and help from others. It is not possible for a person to exist or grow alone. There are only persons in relation. We shape each other's characters and expand or limit their opportunity for growth through social interaction in real time, all the time. People have an inherent need to belong and this requires frequent positive interactions with the same individuals and engagement in these interactions within a framework of long-term, stable care and concern.

In her book, *Seven and a Half Lessons About the Brain*, which I highly recommend, Professor Lisa Feldman Barrett, a renowned American neuroscientist and psychologist sets out to inform readers, "how that three-pound blob between your ears makes you human." She has a lesson devoted to "how your brain secretly works with other brains," in which she points out that humans are a social species and that part of being a social species, it turns out, is that our brains regulate one another's body budgets, namely, the ways bodily resources are used every day. After caregivers have helped their babies to budget their resources efficiently (or badly in the case of Romanian orphans mentioned earlier) and as those little brains wire themselves to their world till their brains are fully grown, they will make deposits of sorts into other people's body budgets as well as make withdrawals too and others do the same to them. She goes on to comment-

"We live longer if we have close, supportive relationships with other people. It may seem obvious that loving relationships are good for us, but studies show that the benefits go beyond what common sense would suggest. If you and your partner feel that your relationship is intimate and caring, that you're responsive to each other's needs, and that life seems easy and enjoyable when you're together, both of you are less likely to get sick. If you're already sick with a serious illness, like cancer or heart disease, you're more likely to get better...............................

...................................Humans are unique in the animal kingdom, however, because we regulate others with *words.* A kind word can calm you, as when a friend gives you a compliment at the end of the day. A hateful word from a bully may cause your brain to predict threat and flood your bloodstream with hormones, squandering precious resources from your body budget."

All of which does not support the maxim, "Sticks and stones will break my bones, but names will never hurt me."

I had the privilege of being mentored, as far as psychology was concerned, by Dr. William E. Hall between 1st August 1991 until his death on 18ᵗʰ April 1998. While he talked about casual or work-a-day relationships and experimental relationships he focused mainly on engaging in exploratory and investment relationships with others. He saw exploratory relationships as an opportunity for people to gradually reveal some of the mystery of their personality and gain an understanding of some of the mystery of another person's personality and enable people to decide what sort of relationship is appropriate between them in the future: should it be one that is close and intimate and worth investing in or one that is more remote and cautious.

For him, essentially exploratory relationships require politely giving others, attention, time and a listening ear and involve the following stages:

(a) giving people attention is critical. Dr. Hall dropped everything and totally focused on others when in the company of others. People would say he made them feel like one in a million. When I was studying him in detail I recall after a meeting of eight people, that all of them stated that Dr. Hall was doing well and making an impact. Yet, he did not say a word during the meeting. I assume that they thought he was giving people approval as they knew he would speak out if he wanted further discussion.

(b) establishing the name by which the person likes to be called, and if it is unusual how to pronounce and spell it and establish if it has a meaning and how it was chosen,

(c) discovering the other person's interests, values and specific goals to see whether any of them are held in common with his own or with the views of others,

(d) talking to them about their talents and strengths, thus seeing the best of them: and finally,

(e) establishing whether the person is trustworthy and ready to enter into an investment relationship.

Usually, he started his exploratory conversations with facts and small talk before asking for opinions as he realized that he wanted people to be comfortable and safe before moving into more vulnerable areas. He maintained, like Voltaire, that, "the best way to the heart is through the ear."

For Dr. Hall, an investment relationship requires at least three people (see Figure.1). Person A uses his/her human relationship capital (mainly consisting of people skills such as empathy, persuasion, openness, integrity, trustworthiness and humility) to bring out the best in person B by getting person B to use his/her human relationship capital to bring out the best in person C.

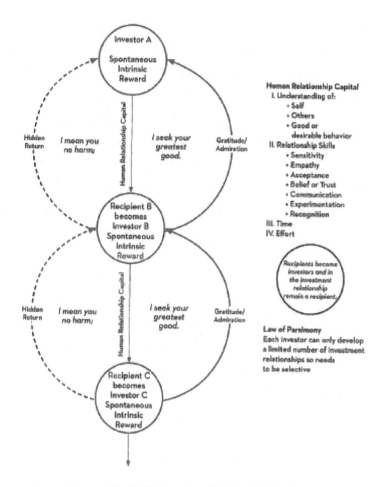

The figure contains the following labels:

Investor A
Spontaneous Intrinsic Reward

Human Relationship Capital
I. Understanding of:
+ Self
+ Others
+ Good or desirable behavior
II. Relationship Skills
+ Sensitivity
+ Empathy
+ Acceptance
+ Belief or Trust
+ Communication
+ Experimentation
+ Recognition
III. Time
IV. Effort

Hidden Return | I mean you no harm; | I seek your greatest good. | Gratitude/ Admiration

Human Relationship Capital

Recipient B becomes Investor B Spontaneous Intrinsic Reward

Recipients become investors and in the investment relationship remain a recipient.

Hidden Return | I mean you no harm; | I seek your greatest good. | Gratitude/ Admiration

Human Relationship Capital

Law of Parsimony
Each investor can only develop a limited number of investment relationships so needs to be selective

Recipient C becomes Investor C Spontaneous Intrinsic Reward

Figure 1. Dr. Hall's Investment Relationship Process.

This process creates a chain-reaction that Dr. Hall called *the ripple effect* which brings out the best in teams, communities and society as a whole. While Dr. Hall worked as the Professor of Educational Psychology and Measurements at the University of Lincoln, Nebraska and later when he became a senior leadership consultant in the business world, he found that when he matched top performers with other people who had high human potential, he obtained his best results. His work on investment relationships emphasised the connectedness of people to each other and stated that when person A actually helps person B for that person's sake, person A always receives a hidden return. By helping you I am in reality helping myself! We are in some way one.

The psychologists Clyde Kluckhohn and Henry A. Murray stated "Every man is in certain respects (a) like all other men, (b) like some other men, and (c) like no other men." To which Dr. Hall would add, "all at the same time."

Statement (a) above is reflected in what I call the **silver rule of good relationships**- "do no harm" which is based on the Hippocratic oath and statement (a) is also based on the **golden rule of good relationship**s- "treat others the way you would like to be treated," which works to a large extent because we are all of the same species, *homo-sapiens*.

Statements (b) and (c) above relate to what I call the **platinum rule of good relationships**- "treat others the way they want or need to be treated," which requires the use of empathy to get to know the uniqueness of each person which at times in their development requires tough love or strict discipline. This rule is also based on one of Dr. Hall's personality themes or typical ways of thinking, feeling or behaving towards others. He called it the 'Individualized Approach' personality theme.

So, my number one recommendation to anyone who wants to live a more fulfilling life and overcome life's challenges, is to surround themselves with, and reach out to trustworthy, compassionate and kind people and never underestimate the healing power of good human relationships. Good relationships build: bad relationships break. When people harm or destroy others the first person they harm or destroy is themselves. Dr. Hall used to say that if you find yourself in a bad human relationship which you cannot change then get out of it as it will gradually destroy you. Good human relationships require humility as the key to opening someone's heart is on the inside and cannot be forced from the outside. Humility is not thinking less of yourself but of thinking of yourself less.

To illustrate the healing power of good relationships I include the following anecdote which involves my working relationship with Dr. Hall. After I had been working with Dr. Hall for a couple of months people started asking me what I was doing to Dr. Hall. "Hold on a minute," I protested, "Don't you mean, what is Dr. Hall doing to me? He is totally changing my perspective on people. So, what precisely are you talking about!" They told me that since Dr. Hall starting working with me, colour had returned to his cheeks, he was walking more upright, there was more bounce in his step and he was more exuberant.

On further consideration I realized that our relationship was mutually beneficial. Previously, I had read and heard about the transformational power of relationships. However, I had a theoretical understanding or an academic grasp of the subject. Now I was actually experiencing the benefits derived from being in a good relationship. I began reflecting on other relationships in my life and noticed how they changed me and the parties involved. Dr. Hall's quote at the beginning of the chapter states that we tend to take human relationships for granted and fail to reflect upon them enough. We are our histories. Memories of others still impact us. People often ask what someone who has died would have done in a particular situation. I suddenly realized the power of good human relationships to help people to become more fully alive, not just mentally but physically and emotionally and that experience was very deep. Dr. Hall recommended that people daily take stock of the vitality of each of their key relationships and take action to further enhance them.

For a more detailed explanation of Dr. Hall's theory and practice please refer to my tribute to his life and work- *Hallways to Success and Significance: The positive Force of Dr. William E. Hall* (2013). In it I explained how Dr. Hall invited people to become significant and successful and I encouraged people to respond to his invitation by following the acronym **R.S.V.P.** by

> **R** - building good relationships with self and others
> **S** - focusing on their own strengths and the strengths of others
> **V** - being vision, values and virtue driven

and by **P** - adopting a positive approach.

Dr. Hall also asked me to identify the attitudes that were essential to all good human relationships, namely trust. I came to the conclusion that if parties to a good human relationship could make two five word promises to each other, then, mutual trust would follow. The two promises are- I mean you no harm; I seek your greatest good. So many people asked me where the ten words came from that I wrote a book to clarify my position, entitled, *I Mean You No Harm; I Seek Your Greatest Good- Reflections on Trust* (April 2015) and slightly revised in March 2023), which also includes further details of my mentor and role model Dr. Hall.

Finally, I would like to bring to your attention some of the latest psychological research from around the world which suggests that stable, healthy, friendships are crucial for our well-being and longevity.

i) People who have friends and close confidants are more satisfied with their lives and less likely to suffer from depression and they are also less likely to die from all causes, including heart problems and a range of chronic diseases.

ii) When people are low in social connection - because of isolation or because of poor quality relationships – they are twice as likely to die prematurely – a risk factor even greater than the effects of smoking 20 cigarettes per day.

iii) Blood pressure reactivity is lower when people talk to a supportive friend rather than a friend whom they feel ambivalent about.

iv) A review of 38 studies found that friendships, especially high-quality ones that provide social support and companionship, significantly predict well-being and can protect against mental health issues such as depression and anxiety – and those benefits persist across the life span.

v) Interactions with acquaintances – and even strangers – can also give our mental health a boost. We learn surprising things when we have unplanned encounters and conversions with people, a benefit that people tend to underestimate.

vi) We can benefit by blurring the lines between Platonic and romantic relationships as there is a symbiosis between them. An analysis of nearly 8,000 respondents to the British Household Panel Survey showed that life satisfaction was about twice as high among people who said that their spouse was also a best friend: marital conflict can trigger unhealthy changes in cortisol levels, but that harm is buffered when spouses feel they have adequate support outside their marriage.

Dr. Hall described a friend as somebody who knows all about you but is still your friend. Making new friendships and making or deepening existing ones takes effort. Recent psychological research in the United States recommends four main steps in creating healthy friendships.

i) Assume people like you

Psychological research on the "liking gap" shows that people tend to underestimate how liked they are when they interact with strangers (Boothey E. J. et al., *Psychological Science*, Vol. 29, No. 11, 2018). When people are told to assume that others like them, they become warmer and friendlier in what's known as the *"acceptance prophecy"* (Stinson D.A. et al., *Personality and Social Psychology Bulletin,* Vol.35, No. 9, 2009).

Rebbecca Scwartz-Mette, PhD, an associate professor of clinical psychology at the University of Maine stated that, "The research suggests that negative thoughts we have about ourselves in social situations may not match with what others are actually thinking about us."

ii) Listen to others

Research by Thalia Wheatley, PhD a psychology professor at Dartmouth College has shown that both friends and strangers feel more connected when their conversationist responds to them quickly *(PNAS,* Vol. 119, No. 4, 2022). "That has to come naturally, through really listening and trying to get what the person is saying. There's no easy hack for friendship- it's just caring enough to listen to each other.

iii) Be consistent

Julianne Holt-Lunstad, PhD, a professor of neuroscience at Brigham Young University sees social activity being similar to physical activity and states that, "You can't maintain physical fitness by just exercising once. It requires regular practice, and investing in your relationships also takes time."

iv) Aim for companionship

Companionship is a key characteristic of a high quality and healthy friendship so connecting with people who have similar hobbies, interests, attitudes and values is a good strategy (Ledbetter, A. M., et al., *Personal Relationships,* Vol. 14, No.2,2007).

One of the main themes of the next chapter on the brain's role in pain creation and relief, is that the person providing the treatment has a huge impact on the outcomes experienced by the person receiving the treatment. For instance, positive words and suggestions by a carer can relieve pain and negative words can create anxiety and increase pain. If a person in pain believes in the healer and has confidence in the effectiveness of the healer's approach then pain relief will result. Effective healers foster a relationship of trust and informed confidence and the reduction of anxiety.

Nor should we forget the power of hearty laughter in contributing to our well-being. Dr. Michael Mosley a British journalist reveals how a good belly-laugh reduces pain, boosts our memory and keeps our blood vessels healthy. He states:

"Laughter is the best medicine. Laughter increases your uptake of oxygen rich air, stimulates your heart, lungs and muscles and increases the release of endorphins, also known as the 'feel-good' hormones which promote social bonding. Studies show that people who share a laugh over a funny video like each other more and have a better sense of connection with each other..........A few years ago researchers from

Oxford University measured the pain tolerance of a number of volunteers and gave one group a funny video to watch while another group were given a boring video about golf. They found that those who had belly laughs increased their pain tolerance by 10% while those who tittered or watched golf remained the same........Finally a large study of over 20,000 men and women in Japan who laughed every day were 20% less likely to suffer a heart attack than those who said that they rarely laughed or never laughed at all."

During the radio show Dr. Mosley also spoke to Professor Michael Miller from Pennsylvania University a cardiologist and expert in heart health. He explained that his early research indicated that emotional and mental stress were high risk factors leading to heart attacks and so he decided to study how an opposite factor, laughter would have on heart health. In one major study he showed his volunteers a clip of the movie "Saving Private Ryan," promoting stress and found that their blood vessels constricted. On another date he gave the same volunteers funny clips designed to get them to laugh heartily and in this case the blood vessels opened up, providing them with better vascular health. A few minutes after a belly laugh their blood vessels dilated and the benefits lasted up to twenty-four hours. He explained that the mechanism that took place involved the brain cross-talking with the heart. The brain releases endorphins when we belly laugh which interact with receptors on the endothelium which in turn release nitric oxide which in turn opens the blood vessels at the same time lowering blood pressure and reducing inflammation reducing platelets and lowering cholesterol. His tips for having a healthy heart are a) to reduce emotional and mental stress b) to eat a healthy diet, c) to exercise frequently and d) have a daily belly laugh.

Throughout my life I have felt the benefits of laughing. Many people used to say that you needed to be a comedian to live in Liverpool after the second World War. My maternal great grandfather used to tell stories at family get-togethers. One such story was that as a child he was so poor that his family kept a pig in the corner as an air- freshener; another was that the only thing he was left in a will was a debt! For my wedding my maternal grandfather gave me a white stick because he said I was joining the institute for the blind. Often when mountain-walking I found that telling and hearing jokes boosted the walker's energy levels. Each of my mentors had a great sense of humour and enjoyed the funny side of life. Dr Hall sometimes opened his talks by saying that every Tom, Dick and Harry called him Bill.

My father had an infectious laugh and took me to the Coventry Hippodrome in August 1952 to see Stan Laurel and Oliver Hardy. I only laughed because he enjoyed them so much that they brought tears to his eyes and to the people surrounding him. However, slap-stick has never appealed to me as it involved people being harmed in some way. My father only had to see Tommy Cooper, a famous U.K. comedian and he would burst into laughter! He also used to use humour to help soften bad news. I recall asking him if I could stay up late to listen to the radio as I could not sleep but he took me up to the bedroom and told me that if I slept on the end of the bed I would soon drop off!

In his highly entertaining and erudite book *Humanology - A Scientist's Guide to Our Amazing Existence,* Professor Luke O'Neil (2018) devotes a chapter covering the healing benefits of mirthful laughter, the type where our bellies vibrate. He mentions an experiment which required 33 women to watch *When Harry Met Sally,* a humourus film, who each had monitors attached to their abdomens to measure movements in their bellies. The researchers also measured their natural killer (NK) cells, which are important for the immune system to fight viruses. At a later date the same women watched a dull tourist video.

When watching *Harry Met Sally* there was an average of 30 belly laughs and the NK cell activity was enhanced, indicating a boost in the immune system, whereas watching the Tourist video resulted in one belly laugh on average and little change to the level of NK cells. Professor O'Neil states, "Perhaps it's a good idea for your doctor to prescribe you two tickets to see Dara O'Briain" (A famous Irish comedian).

His chapter makes reference to many studies showing that hearty laughter provides health benefits. One showed that laughing 100 times was the equivalent of 10 minutes on a rowing machine or 15 minutes cycling. Of particular interest to me was a study that showed that laughing can lower blood sugar levels. People with type II diabetes ate a meal and then attended a boring lecture. The next day the same people ate the same meal but then went to a comedy show. Scientists found that having a good laugh kept their blood sugar levels lower than they did after attending the boring lecture.

Professor O'Neil has found that the most convincing scientific work of laughter is its role in improving interpersonal skills and social bonding and quotes the great comedian Victor Borges, who said, "Laughter is the shortest distance between people."

He also describes a scientific attempt to find the world's funniest joke. Out of the thousands of submissions which were rated by 1.5 million people one joke emerged as the winner:-

Two guys go on a hunting trip. One of them collapses, not breathing, skin turning blue.

The other guy calls emergency services and says, "You've got to help me! My friend has collapsed and appears to be dead."

The emergency services say, "Calm down. We can help. First let's make sure he's dead."

There's silence, followed by a gun shot.

The guy gets back on the line and says, "OK! What do we do now?"

Spike Milligan.
The Goon Show
1951

Spike Milligan was one of my favourite comedians who certainly got the last laugh. When he died in 2002, his tombstone was engraved with the epithet, "I told you I was ill."

While Sylvia Plath stated that "Love set you going," from my experience "Love keeps you going," and I expressed these sentiments in the following poem:-

Beyond Loving
Beyond loving there is no greater thing we can do.
When we're through loving, we're through.

Yes. I believe in the healing power of love!

Let us now explore the brain's role in pain creation and relief.

STEP TWO

UNDERSTANDING THE BRAIN'S ROLE IN PAIN CREATION AND RELIEF

"EVERYTHING WE THINK we know about pain is wrong. That's quite a bold statement. But, by and large, it's true. By 'we', I mean us as a society; I mean most people in and outside the medical establishment. We misunderstand the nature of pain and this misunderstanding is ruining the lives of millions."

The Painful Truth
The new science of why we hurt and how we can heal.

Dr. Monty Lyman 2021.

Over the past four and a half years, as previously mentioned, I have experienced much pain, from modest to excruciating in intensity, and ranging from various forms of physical pain resulting from tissue damage, (the most serious of which were the two amputations), to nervous pain, such as diabetic neuropathy and critical limb ischemia. The latter often involved what is termed 'rest-pain' which can be quite severe. This occurred when I was lying on my back in bed and blood was not flowing to heal the wounds in my feet. Accordingly, I had to dangle my legs over the end of the bed and let gravity do the rest (pardon the pun).

As soon as I was told by Mrs. Rachel Sam that it was highly likely that my left leg would need to be amputated, I began finding out what were the likely outcomes of the process and if there was anything I could do to prevent any post-operative pain. As previously mentioned, before I ran my first full marathon race, I read about the need to build up enough glycogen to avoid 'hitting the wall,' so I decided to do some research into the pain of amputees. A number of amputees told me that one of the worst pains to deal with was that coming from the amputated limb itself, especially having an 'itch' coming from the limb which they could not scratch.

During my research I came across Dr. Monty Lyman's book on pain which addressed the question of phantom limb pain and why it occurred and how it could be prevented or healed. As a result of adopting some of his teachings about ensuring that my brain needed to be convinced that my leg had been successfully removed and that the wounds had fully healed, I have never experienced phantom limb pain in either leg. Another factor which may have helped in this regard, was my diabetic neuropathy which is an inability to feel some pain because of damage to certain nerve endings; for instance, when nurses used pins to prick the skin of my feet or when I was exerting aerobic pressure on a treadmill and could not feel chest pain when my blood pressure was exceedingly high. My brain was unaware of the total intensity of any pain in the wounds on my stumps but I made it fully aware that my legs had been successfully removed. Every day, because of my diabetic neuropathy, I inspect the wounds and adjacent skin on my stumps for evidence of blistering so that I can take appropriate remedial action.

I learned that Dr. Lyman's *first painful truth* is, **"injury is neither necessary nor sufficient for pain".** He tells a story about a builder who jumped off a scaffold onto a plank which had a four-inch nail protruding from it which went straight through his boot. When admitted to the Accident & Emergency department of the local hospital he was in so much pain he was given fentanyl, a pain reliever which is one hundred times stronger than morphine. However, when the medical team carefully removed his boot they found that the nail had penetrated between his toes causing no tissue damage whatsoever!

I also learned that Dr. Lyman's _**painful**_ **untruth is that pain is produced in the body and detected by the brain.**

Modern science has demonstrated that the brain creates pain and the truth is that it is the brain's main role is to **protect a body part or system**. Moreover, modern science reveals that there is no single pain centre in the brain. In other words, as Dr. Lyman puts it, "pain is a decision made by the brain-the vast majority of which is outside our conscious control - to tell our conscious mind we are in danger." Pain therefore is a construct of the brain.

Modern neuroscientists like Professor Lisa Feldman Barrett and Professor Anil Seth have come to the conclusion that the brain has to predict what is happening within and outside our bodies and that the brain is not always correct as we know from our illusions and hallucinations and indeed from phantom-limb pain. Often the brain is an over-protector of the body which accounts for the fact that in twenty percent of people experiencing persistent pain (which lasts longer than three months) doctors can find no evidence of any damaged tissue, as the initial tissue that gave rise to pain has already healed, but the patient's brain does not think so. They see the main role of the brain is to balance the body's budget of resources required for survival.

Distraction has been found to be a powerful pain reliever

which we can all use to good effect. When we become so voluntarily engrossed in a task to accomplish something difficult, but worthwhile, we experience a position termed 'flow' by the positive psychologist, Mihaly Csikszentmihalyi, and lose a sense of time, even the need for food and, from my experience, lose a sense of pain. When exposing people to a painful stimulus, like giving them an injection, doctors and nurses can relieve their patients' pain by quizzing their memory or asking about a recent pleasurable experience. Accordingly, we need to engage in activities that distract us from pain, whether it is music, art, writing or meeting friends and encourage others who are in pain, particularly persistent pain, to do likewise.

Another phenomenon which demonstrates that the brain relieves or increases pain is the **'expectation effect'** otherwise known as the **placebo effect**, (from the Latin, "I shall please") or the **nocebo effect**, (from the Latin, "I shall harm") both of which are responses our brain makes to the **context** in which treatments are delivered. Experiments show that people with positive expectations, self-belief and hope, gain pain relief while people with pessimistic expectations only increase their pain. Scientists discovered that the brain of a person with positive expectations actually releases its own body's opioids such as endorphins, (non-addictive morphine), and other natural painkillers such as dopamine- a molecule associated with pleasure and positive motivation. What we believe, what we remember and what we expect can enable the brain to release the patients' natural painkillers.

As mentioned in the previous part of the book Dr. Lyman

states, "What is becoming increasingly more evident is that the person giving the treatment has a huge impact on the pain relief of the person receiving it." This only underlines the importance of human trust in the healing process. Positive words and suggestions have a positive effect on pain relief.

While the placebo effect generally works at a subconscious level and recipients usually are unaware of being given a placebo, recent scientific studies have shown that even when people are told that they are receiving a placebo the brain still relieves pain. It could be that the recipient really trusts the caregiver and/or is open-minded. Yet the brain is convinced and releases opioids from the body's natural pharmacy. I realise that I am guilty of some repetition here but take consolation from one of my many mentors who stated boldly that if something is worth saying in the first place, then it is worth repeating!

What follows are some anecdotes and some scientific, evidence-based studies which explain the placebo and nocebo effects.

Dr. Lyman tells of a radio producer who had a lot of pain over many years from fibromyalgia. He had heard of the effectiveness of an electric simulation machine. Accordingly, he acquired one. During an interview on *Airing Pain* he described how fantastic it was initially at relieving his pain and relaxing him. Then he added, "After three months I found that I hadn't plugged it in." His brain was so convinced that the device was effective that it released natural painkillers from his body's pharmacy to relieve his pain. This is a perfect illustration of the placebo effect.

The placebo effect has been around for centuries. Thomas Jefferson, the third American President, writing to a friend in 1807, stated, "One of the most successful physicians I have ever known has assured me that he used more bread pills, drops of colored water and hickory ashes than all other medicines put together."

Since Jefferson's time there has been much skepticism about the practice - doctors using the treatments were called quacks and their patients were often called hypochondriacs or malingerers. However, during the World War II an American anaesthesiologist, Henry Beecher, showed a scientific interest in the phenomenon. He had to treat soldiers in Europe with massive wounds but observed that 32% reported feeling no pain at all, while a further 44% experienced only moderate or slight pain. When given the chance, 75% of them refused the option of taking pain relieving drugs. The soldiers were neither hypochondriacs nor malingerers. When morphine was in short supply, nurses would inject wounded soldiers with a saline solution while assuring them that it was a painkiller. Beecher estimated that the placebo was about 90% as effective as the real drug.

After the war Beecher saw the opposite effect in the civilians in Boston, Massachusetts who had been severely injured in car crashes or industrial accidents. 70% of the patients wanted painkillers. Beecher concluded that the only difference between the soldiers in Europe and the civilians in Boston was the meaning they attached to the context they were in. When soldiers in Europe arrived in a hospital they had moved from a place of danger to a place of safety, because they would be shipped home. Whereas the civilians in Boston had moved from a place of safety into a place of danger, so their brains naturally created pain.

By the 1970s in America all drugs would have to perform better than a placebo to be approved! In drug trials and in most research studies on the efficacy of the placebo effect both the doctors and the patients were totally 'bind' or unaware who had been given the real drug or treatment or the placebo.

However, researchers began adopting an open and honest policy even by labelling the placebo. For instance, in his comprehensive book, *The Expectation Effect,* (2022) David Robson describes the work of Dr. Claudia Carvalho in a public hospital in Lisbon, Portugal. In 2016 she gave her patients suffering with chronic back pain a bottle clearly marked "placebo pills to be taken twice a day," containing orange gelatine capsules. She explained that the pills had no active ingredients, but they could have powerful effects on the body such as conditioning and showed them a video reinforcing her message. She stressed that they did not have to experience an optimistic mood but merely take the pills regularly. Three weeks later participants reported a 30% reduction in their pain scores which was what would be expected by an active drug in treatment. In a follow up paper published in 2020 Carvalho showed that these benefits had continued for five years after the original trial.

On this issue Dr. Monty Lyman focuses on the work of Dr. Ted Kaptchuk, Professor of Medicine at Harvard who is also a pioneer in the 'open – label' placebo effect. He concluded that it wasn't the treatments he gave his patients that relieved their pain but the strong belief that they had in him. In 2010 he carried out an experiment on sufferers of irritable bowel syndrome (IBS). He randomly split IBS sufferers into two groups. The first group had a pleasant conversation but were given no treatment. The second group were given a placebo pill and were told, "Placebo pills made of an inert substance, like sugar pills, have been shown in clinical studies to produce significant improvement in IBS symptoms through mind-body self-healing processes." The second group showed greater improvements than the first group! Such studies offer the prospects of healing therapies that avoid the use of addictive opioids. However, the precise understanding of what is happening in the open-label placebo effect is a complicated process which combines aspects of the brain as a predictive machine when it comes to its perception of reality and its evaluation of the total context and also of the brain's memories of what it is like to feel safe and secure and recall the body's experience of pain reduction.

On the other hand, it has also been found that that some people when taking inert substances or fake treatments fail to experience little or no pain relief or indeed feel greater pain. They experience the nocebo effect. Even Henry Beecher in his paper on the placebo effect reported that some patients receiving dummy pills often experienced symptoms such as nausea, headache, dry mouth, fatigue and drowsiness. Six decades later a team of researchers from Oxford, Cardiff and London in 2016/17 analyzed the data of more than 1,200 placebo-controlled trials and found that half the people receiving the dummy pill reported at least one adverse event in the average trial. In 5% of cases reactions were so severe that the participants discontinued treatment altogether. Such studies suggested a highly specific link to the to the warnings of possible side effects by doctors and drug companies.

Positive expectations can trigger the natural release of dopamine and opioids and relieve pain whereas negative expectations deactivate these same neurotransmitters. In addition, negative expectations can trigger the release of cholecystokinin (CCK), which boosts the transmission of pain signals. Based on its expectations the brain will also instruct the nervous, immune, circulatory and digestive systems in certain ways that could result in inflammation, altered blood pressure, nausea and the release of hormones that would increase stress levels. Since the brain draws on its memories to predict its responses the chances of experiencing a nocebo side effect based on the one you have just had become more likely in the future. It is quite difficult to forget food we have eaten which made us ill.

One thing we know is, that it is possible to change our expectations, develop a more positive mindset and live a happier and healthier life. There are certain skills we can practice that can reframe the way we see the world, especially when it comes to the world of pain. For instance, when considering the side-effects of certain drugs which are advertised as being ineffective for 15% of patients treated, we can reframe the advert to read that 85% of patients will be free from adverse symptoms.

We can also reappraise the actual pain we suffer. Some people have a tendency to exaggerate or worry about any painful experience they have had rather than trying to find out whether it is indeed evidence of a temporary healing side effect. I recall a story about an American Indian Chief who told his fellow tribesmen that inside every warrior there exist a negative and positive fighting force competing to gain control. When the Chief was asked which force won in his case, he said the one that he fed the most!

The power of the brain has been underestimated throughout the ages because it occupies only about 2 percent of the body and looks like a three-pound blob of grey gelatin. Indeed, the ancient Egyptians saw it as a useless organ not worth preserving and pulled it out through the noses of dead pharaohs! Generally, throughout history it was regarded as merely responding to stimuli. Relatively recently it has been recognized as an ever-active organ containing 86 billion neurons. An organ, which from behind a skull, proactively predicts almost everything human beings do, rather than being triggered like a reflex. The brain's main function is to ensure that the body survives and is safe and secure.

The brain tries to make sense of the external sensations it receives from the external environment and the internal sensations it receives from the body and if it predicts there is damage to the body it will to do whatsoever it takes to protect the body, releasing endorphins to relieve pain. If it predicts that an organ or system is in serious danger it will activate pain systems that alert the body to take any appropriate protective actions.

Recently there was a pain pandemic in the United States between 2019 and 2021 where persistent pain was treated with opioids. Opioids are very effective for short term pain but are much less affective for persistent pain and they become addictive, with larger doses needed to provide the same relief. People on long term opioids often develop dependence, that is, they need to have the drug to maintain normal functions and exhibit severe negative withdrawal symptoms if taken off them too quickly. To make things worse taking opioids over a long period of time can increase sensitivity to pain. Major pharmaceutical companies have created synthetic opioids like OxcyContin and fentanyl. During the persistent pain pandemic doctors were given incentives to prescribe them for all sorts of pain which led to hundreds of thousands opioid overdose deaths and suicides.

What then are the main reasons why pain persists after the original tissue that gave rise to the pain has healed or in other words why does pain remain after healing has occurred?

In short, the brain becomes more sensitive to any changes in the area where the original tissue damaged occurred. The brain begins to misinterpret what is actually is going on in the tissues. There is a false alarm. Now there is pain with less sensitivity than actually occurred in the first place. Even though the tissue damage has completely healed, a pain 'memory' exists in the brain. Brain networks which are activated frequently become stronger and those activated less frequently become underused or fade into insignificance. The protective brain is now overacting to sensations it is receiving; in other words, the central nervous system becomes over sensitive. As we shall see later the brain needs to become rewired and use its neuroplasticity more efficiently.

It is interesting to note that roughly three quarters of persistent-pain sufferers experience sleep disturbance and half of individuals with insomnia have persistent pain. An issue we will address in the next part of the book.

STEP THREE

USING THE RESTORATIVE POWER OF SOUND SLEEP

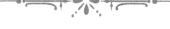

"I wake to sleep, and take my waking slow.
I feel my fate in what I cannot fear.
I learn by going where I have to go."

The Waking,
Theodore Roethke
1953

The Waking is one of the most beautiful and enigmatic poems I have ever read. Roethke, an American poet, uses the rigid structure of the French villanelle to express his thoughts and feelings, as did Dylan Thomas in his iconic poem "Do Not Go Gentle Into That Good Night." For Roethke, the title is a metaphor for a person's conscious life. He takes his readers on a journey from birth through different stages of consciousness to the final sleep, that is death. He hints that he takes his waking slow, not because of cautious fear, but because he savours life, something he wants to prolong and enjoy and at the same time learn in which direction to go.

It reminds me of a diagram in Professor Anil Seth's book, *Being You- A New Science of Consciousness* (see Figure. 2). Seth states," For each of us our conscious experience is *all there is*. Without it there is nothing at all: no world, no self, no interior and no exterior." In his book Seth attempts, "to understand how the inner universe of subjective experience relates to, and can be explained in terms of biological and physical processes unfolding in brains and bodies."

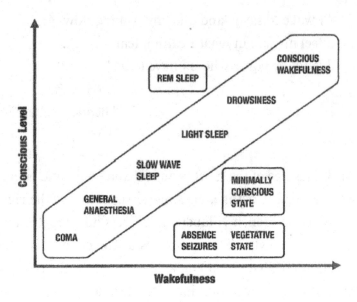

Figure 2. Dr. Anil Seth's diagram of the relation between consious level (awareness) and wakefulness (arousal).

When in a coma or a vegetative state, consciousness is completely absent although there is some minimal trace of electrochemical neural circuitry: there is some light on but nobody is home. When a person is under general anaesthetic the brain's electrical activity is almost entirely cancelled. It is very different from sleep: if a person was just asleep the surgeon's scalpel would quickly wake him or her up. Under a deep anaesthetic a person experiences no pain whatsoever, even when having their legs amputated! When sleeping, people go through 4/5 sleep cycles which include light sleep, deep sleep, rapid eye movement (REM) sleep, when they are having some conscious dreaming experiences. This is followed by a short period of drowsiness and then by full consciousness and wakefulness.

Professor Seth states, "I will make the case that experiences of *being you* and of *being me* emerge from the way the brain predicts and controls the internal state of the body. The essence of selfhood is neither a rational mind nor an immaterial soul. It is a deeply embodied biological *process,* a process that underpins the simple feeling of being alive that is the basis for all our experiences of self, indeed any conscious experience at all. Being you is literally about your body....... Our conscious experiences are part of nature, just as our bodies are and our world is. And when life ends, consciousness will end." For him, consciousness is first and foremost about subjective experience and he is intent on finding ways by which it can be measured.

In my life I was in a comma for 72 hours or so when I was six years old and under general anaesthetic nine times throughout my life for a total of between 35 to 40 hours. From my experience sleep is not always a state of unconscious bliss, especially when dreaming about distressing events, like falling or losing my wallet or passport. In fact, it was often a relief to wake up and be grateful that I had only been dreaming. However, there is nothing worse than being unable to sleep while experiencing severe pain. I recall on many occasions lying awake in bed in severe pain trying to resolve a conundrum - does insomnia cause pain or does pain cause insomnia? For me the jury is still out.

However, reflecting on the teachings of Dr. Lyman, the latest scientific view is that when the brain perceives danger in the body, in this case the inability to get restful sleep, it triggers the pain network to make the body take appropriate action to restore safety and security. Accordingly, insomnia causes more pain than pain causes insomnia. So, what action can we take to make the brain feel safe and secure enough to allow us to fade peacefully into slumber?

Certainly, I have taken prescribed opioids like liquid morphine and codeine after major surgery but I knew that in the long term, they reduce sleep quality and worsen pain. So, I only used them in the very short term, that is for a week or so. Then I used weaker over the counter pain killers like co-codamol and paracetamol to relieve pain so that I could sleep. Sometimes these medications took a lot of time before they took effect or had little or no effect and the pain became so severe that I just passed out.

Most neuroscientists agree that bodily energy efficiency is key to human survival and that the brain acts as a command centre when it comes to controlling the human body's resources. Lisa Feldmann Barrett states, "You can think about energy efficiency like a budget……. A budget for your body which tracks water, salt and glucose as you gain and lose them…. Your brain is guessing when to spend resources and when to save them…………………prediction beats reaction. The scientific name for body budgeting is allostasis."

Let us examine some key aspects of the science of how sleeping well will enhance or replenish our body energy budget.

Everybody needs sleep which carries out a number of different functions, including cleaning the brain of toxins, physical restoration, improving information processing and memorisation, regulating moods and strengthening the immune system all of which are restorative functions.

In July 2023 a documentary on British TV called "Sleep Well...Live Better," claimed that in England 74% of people have trouble sleeping at least sometimes and that 39% often or always had difficulty sleeping. A poll of 2,209 adults led researchers to estimate that one in ten people experienced chronic insomnia (which lasts three months or more). The programme also stated that insufficient sleep costs the UK economy £40 billion in terms of lost Gross Domestic Product (GDP). Sleep deprivation levels in the United States according to the Center for Disease Control (CDC) maintain that 1 in 3 people consider that they do not receive adequate sleep or rest daily.

It is essential for the brain to feel safe and secure to enable the body to relax and fall asleep and for adults to get quality sleep daily in accordance with our in-built body clock, known as our *circadian rhythm*. Professor Luke O'Neil describes a typical body clock day as follows:-

"Most adults wake between 6am and 9am when testosterone peaks to get us ready for the activities that face us. Between 9am and 12noon our cortisol peaks which gives our brains a boost of alertness. We tend to be most productive at work before lunch, when our short - term memory is at its best. Our body makes digestive enzymes in anticipation of eating and we feel hungry because of the release of hormones such as ghrelin, which stimulates the parts of our brain that then say 'you're hungry'. Between 12noon and 3pm our bodies will be full of food.

And, of course, once we've eaten, we experience that early-afternoon slump, the post-lunch dip. Our alertness takes a nose – dive at this time................Between 3pm and 6pm our body temperature rises slightly, our hearts and lungs work better and our muscles are 6 percent stronger.....Between 6pm and 9pm you are ready for dinner. However, don't leave this too late...... as we are likely to store food as fat...one useful thing, though, is our liver can break down alcohol at this time, so now is the safest time to drink. From 9pm to midnight, bedtime is looming.... Our bodies make our own sleeping tablet in the form of melatonin. When our eyes detect dimming light, melatonin is secreted by the pineal gland in our brains and makes us fall asleep....... Blue light suppresses its production and is the wavelength of light emitted from computers and smart phones .... melatonin gets made earlier if you are a morning lark or later if you are a night owl......... From midnight to 3am you are asleep, and the sluice gates open to flush out the debris from your brain that has built up during the day.............From 3am to 6am hopefully you are still asleep, but melatonin levels start to fall to get you ready to wake up........It has recently been shown that our immune systems are more active at night than during the day....... Rheumatoid arthritis is a disease where our immune system attacks our bodies. It's worse at night,....."

Throughout the day and especially towards the end of the day I focus on helping my brain feel safe and secure in my body by being mindful and knowing that I cannot change the past and regard the future as a time to make a positive difference and take new initiatives. Breathing deeply and exhaling slowly helps me to relax and focus on the present.

On the 2nd January 2024 I listened to a radio discussion between Dr. Michael Mosely and Russell Foster, Professor of the Sleep and Circadian Neuroscience Institute at Oxford University who is a world leader when it comes to understanding what makes our biological body clocks tick.

Initially they discussed the link between the circadian system and sleep before Mosley asked Foster. what he regarded to be his five top tips to help people get a better sleep which are summarized below:-

1. Do not obsess about the mythological need for a continuous block of eight hours sleep every night.

Professor Foster pointed out that this figure is an average and explains that the National Sleep Foundation states that people should sleep for a range of six to ten and a half to eleven hours daily. He maintains that what really matters is what is each individual person's sleep range. Instead, people are suffering sleep anxiety which is keeping them awake worrying about their inability to hit the mythological eight-hour target. He urges people to examine how they feel during the day to see how bright, alert, edgy, grumpy or tired they feel and he encourages them to listen to the comments of others and notice their reactions to them too. By doing this people will be able to establish whether or not they are getting enough sleep. Professor Foster tells of some research of sleep patterns of people prior to the industrial age which found that often it was bimodal or even for some, a polyphasic pattern. After sleeping for several hours most people would wake up and interact with others, do some relaxing things like having sex before returning to bed for several hours of sleep before waking up refreshed. The research also found that certain people had polyphasic sleep patterns involving several blocks of sleep during the night and intervals of relaxation including listening to music or reading etc. Accordingly, when people stop worrying about waking intervals and relax they will become less anxious and sleep better. For him anxiety is the enemy of sound sleep.

2. Make big decisions when you have slept on them.

Professor Foster explained that a good night's sleep improves the decision-making circuitry in the brain. For him, the brain during sleep enjoys playing with data, memories, problems it is trying to solve and making creative matches. The brain, he says, is extremely active while we sleep and has more time available than when awake to explore issues as it has less external bodily sensations to interpret. Indeed, he mentions a research project which involved three stages.

In stage 1 he asked a group to consider and become familiar with a complicated problem throughout the morning and then asked them to solve the problem that afternoon. The success rate was 20%.

In stage 2 he asked another group to spend time considering the same cognitive problem but asked them to solve the problem the next day following a night without any sleep. The success rate was again 20%.

In stage 3 he asked another group to spend time considering the same problem and to solve the problem the following afternoon after a good night's sleep. This time the success rate was 60-70%.

Dr. Mosley then asked him whether people make breakthroughs during their sleep and he mentioned several, including one I can relate to, namely, Sir Paul McCartney's composition of "Yesterday," which was a similar experience I had when composing the poem "Total Mutual Trust," which I describe at the beginning of my book "I Mean You No Harm; I Seek Your Greatest Good - Reflections on Trust."

Professor Foster ends this tip by stating that older adults are more cognitively active between 11.00. am to 12.00 pm and teenagers are more cognitively active between 2.00. pm to 3.00. pm. Which means after a good night's sleep they can make better decisions at these times.

3. Know your chronotype.

Professor Foster explains that there are three types of sleepers: **larks** (approximately 10% of the population) who are early to bed and early to rise, **doves** (approximately 65% of the population) who go to bed around 10 to 11 pm and rise around 7am. in the morning and **night owls** (approximately 25% of the population) who go to sleep after midnight and rise later than larks and doves.

These types of sleepers Foster maintains are the amalgam

of three factors, genetics, age and exposure to light. He encourages people to adapt their chronotypes to fit their lifestyles. A lark can become more of a night owl by gaining more exposure to light later in the day and a night owl can become more of a lark by exposing themselves to natural light earlier in the morning.

4. A great night's sleep starts when you wake up.

Professor Foster states that we are used to thinking that a great night's sleep gives us a better day. However, he sees them as reciprocal. The quality of our awake state gives us a better quality of our sleep state and vice versa.

During the day he encourages people of the benefits of taking a nap providing it is no longer than twenty minutes in duration and not before bedtime. He tells people not to drink caffeine after two in the afternoon as caffeine blocks the build-up of adenosine receptors in the brain which make you feel more awake and alert and under less pressure to sleep. Towards the end of the day he urges people to wind down for a period and relax and sees the benefits of practicing mindfulness or yoga or meditation and avoid taking alcohol three hours before sleep. At least thirty minutes before going to sleep Professor Foster advises people to stop using electronic devices and to attend to matters of sleep hygiene in the bedroom such as keeping the temperature at about eighteen degrees Celsius. For him the bedroom should be somewhere quiet, with reduced light and a haven for sleep or sex and nothing else.

5. Don't have difficult conversations when tired and lying in bed before sleep.

Exchanges concerning financial matters or wills or other potential stressful subjects should be avoided as they can create anxiety, which is an enemy of sound sleep. Foster points out that the tired brain will remember negative experiences and forget positive experiences. The whole world view of a tired brain is biased by a negative salience. People become less empathetic, more impulsive and more irritable. He states that divorce rates for nightshift workers is six times higher when compared with dayshift workers.

Dr. Mosley ends their conversation by asking Professor Foster if he could only choose one tip of the five given what would it be and he replied tip number 4 – a great night's sleep starts when you wake up!

I have found that currently being a night owl, that it is very beneficial for me to go to bed at the same time every night seven days a week. I make sure that my bladder is empty before I get into bed. Once I am in bed and ready to sleep, I find it useful to take deep breaths through my nose and slowly exhale through my mouth which usually enables me to peacefully fade away. Most nights I wake for a short period or two but by using my breathing techniques soon return to sleep perchance to dream. Occasionally, I will remain awake for long periods but I enjoy using that time to address unresolved problems or fine tune ways of expressing ideas. I return to wakefulness around the same time every day and then I enjoy to, "take my waking slow."

5. Don't have difficult conversations when tired and trying [illegible] before sleep.

Exchanges concerning emotional matters or [illegible] or other emotional stressful [illegible] should be avoided as they [illegible] create [illegible], which is an enemy of [illegible]. [illegible] points out that the tired brain will remember negative experiences and forget positive experiences. The whole world view of [illegible] tired brain [illegible] by anxious [illegible] [illegible] more [illegible] [illegible]

[illegible]

[illegible] not [illegible] [illegible] [illegible] sleep.

[illegible]

[illegible] and [illegible] ready [illegible] deep [illegible] my [illegible] and [illegible] exactly the same way. Most nights I [illegible] short [illegible] out [illegible] but the [illegible] percentage of [illegible]. Occasionally, I will remain awake for [illegible]. I enjoy using that time to [illegible] unresolved problems [illegible] of expressing ideas I [illegible] to [illegible] wake [illegible] time [illegible] and then I [illegible] to [illegible] awake [illegible].

STEP FOUR

BUILDING HOPE AND DETERMINATION

"Do all you can with what you've got,
In the time you have,
In the place you are."

Nkosi Johnson

July 2000.

Nkosi Johnson was born HIV-positive on 4th February 1989. These words are attributed to him as having been made during the 13th AIDS conference in Durban, South Africa in July 2000 when he was eleven years old. He was living with full blown AIDs. He died on 1st June 2001 from an AIDs related disease, weighing eighteen pounds, one pound for each word in the quote. In the inaugural address he captured the hearts of millions when he appealed to them to "Care for us and accept us- we are all human beings- we are normal. We have hands. We have feet. We can walk, we can talk, we have needs just like everyone else – don't be afraid of us – we are all the same!"

I first came across this amazing child when I read the book, *We are all the Same* by Jim T. Wooten shortly after it was published in 2004. Nkosi did more than President Mandela to raise the awareness of and the support required for those born HIV positive or were diagnosed with HIV or suffered full blown AIDS in South Africa. His compassionate voice about the plight of people like him reverberated around other African countries and eventually echoed around the globe before he died nearly twenty-three years ago. Even today his courage and his words still stir and inspire people into positive action.

Another person who spent time in Africa courageously

pursuing her dreams was the iconic conservationist, Dr. Jane Goodall. Despite mainstream philosophers and scientists of the time stating that humans were the only animals who had intelligence and were toolmakers she lived with and studied chimpanzees in Gombe and showed that they could intelligently make and use tools and, communicate and express feelings. She went on to become a determined and compassionate conservationist, intent on improving and saving the planet and many of its species.

Towards the end of 2023 Dr. Jane Goodall, appeared as a sitter to have her portrait painted by Wendy Barratt the winner of Sky television's show *Portrait Artist of 2023*. During the show they talked about perseverance, determination and the power of hope during which Dr. Jane Goodall made the following remarks:-

"I see the human race as at the mouth of a very, very long dark tunnel and right at the end is a little star, and that's hope. But we don't sit at the mouth of the tunnel and hope it comes to us. We have to clamber over, crawl under and work our way around all the obstacles that lie between us and hope............. If you lose hope you give up. If people lose hope, they become apathetic. How could you possibly think of all the little children being born into a world where everybody has given up. What a nightmare!............So our *Roots and Shoots* (youth groups), at the end of a meeting where they gather together were saying, together we can save the world, and now they say, together we can save the world and together we will save the world, and I say Yes! because we MUST."

While I was working as a positive psychologist in the

United States I came across the work of another positive psychologist, Charles "Rick" Snyder who was a leading theorist and promoter of human hope. He suggested that what people hope and expect to happen influences their behavior. For him desired and meaningful goals were essential to hope and must require effort to be achieved. Hope lies somewhere between a mindset and a skillset; something we can all keep practicing and developing, rather than something which people have or do not have. He stated that once goals have been set then pathways need to be identified which, when followed, lead to the realization of those goals. Once goals are met the process becomes self-reinforcing and enables people to set more ambitious goals and so the cycle is continued, especially from the acknowledgement they receive from the confidence others have in their ability. Certainly Dr. Hall promoted the power of human recognition to unlock human potential.

Change for the better is a key ingredient in human hope. In her brilliant book *How Emotions Are Made,* Lisa Feldman Barrett provides scientific evidence to support her theory that emotions are constructed by the brain rather than by being automatic reflex reactions triggered by external and internal stimuli received by the brain. She puts a strong case forward for the human being's ability to choose what emotions the person wants to display and feel. For her, adults can choose to educate themselves and learn new concepts and become, in her words, "architects of their own experience" and not the victims of their emotions. She maintains that the brain operates by prediction and construction and wires and rewires itself through experience and claims that is not an overstatement to say, "if you change your current experience today, you can change who you become tomorrow."

She draws a sharp distinction between a person's simple feelings of *affect,* from their instances of more complex emotions.

Affect has two features - of pleasantness or unpleasantness (known as valence) and at the same time being highly intense or extremely calm (known as arousal). Affect is a fundamental aspect of consciousness which never turns off from birth to death. Affect is the result of the brain's representation of all sensations from internal organs and tissues, the hormones in blood, and the immune system (technically known as *interoception*).

In her book she explains how people can master their emotions by keeping their body budgets in balance and in good shape. Starting with eating healthfully, exercising regularly and getting enough quality sleep, for which there is, speaking biologically, no substitute. She then recommends that people become more "emotionally intelligent," by which she means "getting your brain to construct the most useful emotion in a given context or situation. (And also, when *not* to construct emotions but instances of some other concept.)" In this regard, she encourages people to increase the number of emotional concepts they have and become more expert in expressing their emotions more precisely.

Also, on a practical level she helps her readers to understand how emotion and illness are connected. She is of the view that chronic pain, chronic stress, and depression and anxiety are constructed in the same manner as emotions are as far as the predictive brain and the body budget is concerned. A person's brain anticipates the body's needs throughout the day and shifts around the body's budgetary resources like oxygen, glucose, salt and water accordingly. For instance, when digesting food, the brain transfers resources from various muscles and when running, the brain transfers resources from the liver and kidneys to the muscles. Most transfers keep the body budget solvent. However, when the brain estimates incorrectly, the body budget moves out of balance. In general, these imbalances are okay as long as they are corrected. If such imbalances become prolonged and remain uncorrected the body budget goes into the red and can be devasting to a person's health. She concludes that complex illnesses such as chronic pain, chronic stress and autism, like emotions are constructed by the brain and like emotions can be changed for the better. The brain needs to predict accurately to avoid body and mental imbalances such as phantom limb pain and when overprotecting the body by predicting that tissue is damaged when in fact it has healed, resulting in chronic pain. Whenever, the brain thinks that a person is in danger or not secure it releases pain to alert that further remedial action is required. If a person has difficulty getting to sleep the brain will initiate pain. In such cases insomnia results in pain rather than pain resulting in insomnia. For Lisa Feldman Barrett the possibility of change offers people suffering with severe illnesses like chronic pain, severe depression and anxiety and autism a great deal of hope.

Another area that offers hope to amputees is to recall

what has been previously written about the expectation effect and assure ourselves that we can, with effort, change our expectations and live healthier lives.

Finally, I would like to further endorse Dr. Hall's Positive Approach and his sense of realistic optimism. I remember when I first went to work with Dr. Hall on August 1st, 1991 in Atlanta, Georgia in the United States that he had a plaque on his desk containing a copy of The Optimist Creed. I wrote it down and sent a copy to Maureen as it was indicative of a completely different workplace culture to the one I had left in the UK motor Industry. It went as follows:-

The Optimist Creed

Promise yourself
To be so strong that nothing can disturb your peace of mind.
Talk health, happiness and prosperity to every person you meet.
To make all your friends feel that there is something in them.
To look at the sunny side of everything and make your optimism come true.
To think only of the best, to work only for the best, and expect only the the best.
To be just as enthusiastic about the success of others as you are about your own
To forget the mistakes of the past and press on to the greater achievements of the future.
To wear a cheerful countenance at all times and give every living creature you meet a smile.

To give so much time to the improvement of yourself that you
   have no time to criticize others.
To be too large for worry, too noble for anger, too strong for
   fear and too happy to permit the presence of trouble.
Optimist International

Optimism was a key aspect of Dr. Hall's Positive Approach
but he was aware of the need to respond to negativity too. He
realized that what someone stands for, then the opposite they
must be against. He definitely was not a starry-eyed Pollyanna.

In the last chapter of his book- "The Pain Revolution"-
Dr. Lyman sets out what he considers to be the most effective
ways or treatments he has come across to relieve pain. The
first being education, as he puts it, "We cannot re-wire what
we do not understand..... One of the pioneering works in
pain education Is *Explain Pain,* a book and educational course
created by the Australian pain experts (and pain explainers)
David Butler and Lorimer Mosely." He also recommends an
app *Curable* and a book by Dr. Deepak Ravindran- "The Pain
Free Mindset*" in which he uses the acronym **MINDSET** as
a mnemonic,

   M for Medications
   I for Interventions
   N for neuroscience education
   D for diet
   S for sleep
   E for exercise
   T for therapies for mind and body

Dr. Lyman also describes a surprise method of relieving pain for many, namely, **Knitting** and makes reference to Betsan Corkhill's book – "Knitting for Health and Wellness." Corkhill also conducted a survey of 3,500 knitters and concluded that 90 per cent of those with persistent pain said that knitting was a successful means of coping with their condition. She says knitting works because it meets the requirements of her equation: knitting = movement + an enriched environment + social engagement.

Finally, Dr. Lyman makes reference to the work of Dr. Michael Moskowitz who is a pain expert who helps people to follow his example of successfully rewiring his brain out of pain after having himself suffered thirteen years of miserable pain. In addition, he touches on the healing powers of sleep, relaxation and breathing properly.

Although I have not taken up knitting, I owe a debt of gratitude to Dr. Lyman in helping me to become free of severe pain, for providing me with coping skills and also for giving me hope that I will be able to manage if I were to suffer severe pain in the future.

In his excellent book *Emotional- The New Thinking About Feelings*, Leonard Mlodinow provides a comprehensive overview of the latest scientific knowledge of the nature of emotions and feelings and how we can manage them and live happier lives. He has a chapter on the meaning of determination. In this chapter he cites many examples of extraordinary determination including the knockout of Mike Tyson by James "Buster" Douglas in Tokyo in February 1990.

In this fight Douglas was knocked down in the eighth-round,

but was saved by the bell. However, he came out fighting and in the final seconds of the tenth round knocked out Tyson, which still stands as the greatest upset in the history of boxing. Mlodinow also includes Roger Bannister's under four-minute mile. In both cases it was as if a mental switch were thrown, namely, a realization that the task could be done, which led to the determination to keep pushing until it was accomplished, in spite of obstacles and challenges.

Mlodinow goes on to explain where determination comes from. He points out that as a species we have a prime directive to survive and a secondary one to seek reward and avoid punishment. Moreover, determination has both a physical component in the brain and a mental component which can be accessed through psychological events. He states, "Losing a loved one changes your brain. So does a pep talk. So does brain surgery. And as we'll see, in the longer term so do exercise and meditation."

In 2007 the neural circuits that govern the physical side of determination were discovered – "the emotional salience network" and the "executive control network." Both networks are distinct but work together. The former monitors our internal emotions and our external environment and decides what is important and the latter has the job of keeping us focused on what is relevant to the achievement of our goals while ignoring distractions.

Mlodinov describes how in 2013 in Stanford Medical School a group of neuroscientists were trying to pinpoint the source of seizures in a patient with severe epilepsy. They implanted electrodes in various areas of the patient's brain and asked about their sensations, thoughts and feelings. They were surprised, on one of the cycles of treatment, a man felt "determination." The feeling wasn't associated with any particular goal; it was just an abstract feeling, a positive feeling that says push harder, push harder, push harder. Inadvertently, the group of neuroscientists had pinpointed the precise anatomical coordinates that support complex psychological and behavioural states associated with perseverance. In 2017 a team of researchers working with rats was able to stimulate their brains to activate a "grit switch" in the emotional salience/executive control complex in order to increase their resilience and determination.

Other than serious cases of human apathy which require stimulation of the emotional salience/executive control complex, Mlodinow states that researchers have found that exercising as little as fifteen minutes a day improves your cardiac fitness, leads to a better executive control system and greater determination. Another way Mlodinow has discovered to increase determination is through mindfulness meditation, which teaches attention control, emotion regulation and increased self-awareness. He cites a study of smokers who undertook two weeks training in mindfulness which led to a 60% reduction in smoking and that brain imaging after the training confirmed a significant increase in activity in the executive control network.

In the final stages of the chapter Mlodinow includes a determination questionnaire developed by psychologists for readers to establish their base level of determination or drive. He also discusses how ageing can have a negative effect on determination and stresses that sleep deprivation, though not an illness nor an injury, has a significant negative effect on determination. He provides strong evidence that sleep provides a nightly recalibration that restores the appropriate emotional salience responses that are necessary to guide appropriate decisions and actions.

In the third and final part of his book Mlodinow helps readers to develop their emotional profile as far as seven emotions are concerned-shame, guilt, anxiety, anger aggression, joy/happiness and romantic love/attachment, which he regards to be the most influential human emotions. He includes seven research validated assessment tools and encourages his readers to complete them and to get significant others in their lives to take them too and compare and discuss them.

In the final chapter of his book Mlodinow focuses on managing emotions which provides his readers with some hope of being able to control emotions instead of becoming victims of them. He provides specific scientific evidence to support the healthy emotional outcomes of three approaches:-

1. **Stoical acceptance of circumstances and focusing on matters that you can control and ignoring and avoiding matters you can't.**

In particular, Stoics like Epictetus, warned about reacting emotionally to what is outside of our control like getting angry with the rain for spoiling our picnic or getting angry with someone who mistreats us as we usually can't control or change this person any more than we can banish rain. Stoics focus on what they can do to make their lives better. Stoics trained themselves to accept and handle adversity and to accept unpleasant thoughts and not to fight them or the feelings they give rise to. "Their triumphs," were, as Mlodinow points out "a classic case of rationality and emotion working together; through brain processes the Stoics might have intuited but could not have explained the executive network structures in our prefrontal cortex exerting influence over the many subcortical structures associated with emotion. When we successfully orchestrate that, we achieve emotional regulation".

Obviously, the Stoics had no idea about individual, community and international responsibility when it comes to climate change and conservation of life globally. However, rather than getting angry with the climate there are always positive actions we can take individually or in groups by peaceful protest or by taking positive action to recycle products, using less plastic, promoting renewable resources, planting more trees and using less oil etc.

2. It is possible to control emotions by re-appraising or putting an alternative spin on the circumstances giving rise to the original emotional assessment or feelings experienced.

Mlodinow states, "Reappraisal involves recognizing the negative pattern developing in your thoughts and changing it to one that is more desirable, but is in a manner that is still based in reality........Research on re-appraisal has shown that we have the power to choose the meanings we assign to circumstances, events and experiences in our lives. Instead of resenting that server who seems to be ignoring you, you can view the server as a victim of too many tables. Instead of viewing the person who is always boasting about how much money he makes as obnoxious, you can view him as insecure because everyone else in your social group has a more interesting job than he does. Even if the negative appraisal won't completely dissipate, the positive alternatives add new possibilities to your thinking, moderating your tendency to look at things in a negative way."

In short, change the stimulus and you will change the response and become more emotionally in control.

3. **Expressing emotions, or using the healing power of words, will enable us to better control our emotions.**

Mlodinow states that recent psychological surveys indicate that most people think that writing or talking about emotions does not help to overcome unwanted emotion and indeed think it only makes our situation worse. However, he finds that clinical psychologists have found that talking is most effective when the sharing is done with friends or a significant other, especially if they have experienced similar issues. Moreover, he provides evidence that talking or writing about emotions lowers the stress felt after viewing disturbing photos or videos, calming the anxiety of people who are nervous about public speaking and reducing the severity of post-traumatic stress disorder. In addition, simply writing about upsetting experiences has been shown to lower high blood pressure, lessen persistent pain symptoms and boost the immune function.

There is also much anecdotal evidence about the positive value of talking or writing about emotions and Mlodinow mentions the experience of a senior executive of a Hollywood production company whose job required her to deal with many difficult people even after they break commitments or treat her unfairly. At times she grows angry and found that used to get in the way she carried out her work. So, she decided to write an email to the offender describing in detail the perceived injustice and openly stating her honest and uncensored feelings about it. But she does not send the email, putting it in her drafts, to send a few days later but never does. She found that the simple process of expressing her feelings has already solved her problems. She soon gets over her debilitating anger and goes back to work.

Mlodinow also described a study in 2019 of a hundred thousand Twitter users which confirmed that expressing their views about their feelings defused their effect.

It is now the end of May 2024 and the Selly Oak Rehabilitation physiotherapy team have agreed that it is safe enough for me to walk using arm-length crutches (see Photo.3). This has increased my mobility enormously and has given me more freedom. I am hoping to further increase my strength and balance so that I can walk aided by waist-length crutches only by the time of my 82nd birthday on 20th September 2024, and who knows, to walk with the use of one waist-length crutch after my right stump is due to finally stabilize in April 2025. At that time, I also hope to become a volunteer coach for the UK Limbless Association. In addition, I have been assessed as having the ability to drive again once controls on my car have been fitted to the steering wheel.

Recently my diabetic medical team have informed me that I am now pre-diabetic and the doctors have halved the medication to reduce my blood glucose levels and will review my blood glucose levels in three months. If my blood glucose levels continue to fall doctors will take me off blood glucose reduction medication altogether and hopefully declare that I have successfully reversed my Type II diabetes. My resolve to stick to my diet and exercise regimen will be critical to achieving this objective.

As I write this ending to the book, I have just heard on the radio that Dr. Michael Mosley is hosting a show providing research which shows that reciting rhyming verse aloud provides significant mental and physical health benefits and helps readers become more hopeful. This makes me think of creating an audio version of the poetry book I wrote for the pandemic, "Armless Hugs," (September 2023) or maybe compiling an anthology of my favourite poems. He has also recently written a book entitled, *4 Weeks to Better Sleep-The science of sleep explored and the secret of a good nights' sleep*, which I am looking forward to reading.

At the moment walking on prosthetic legs is like walking on stilts and involves a great deal of stamina and endurance to cover a small distance but with perseverance and determination I am hoping that it will become easier. I realise that I am no longer a 'spring chicken' and that I will have to face the natural challenges of ageing but the journey I have been on over the last three and a half years and the support I have received from family, friends and professional experts has filled me with confidence and has inspired me to continue in my endeavours.

I am confident that prosthetic leg manufacturers will continue to create more effective and efficient products. Manufacturers of walking aids are also improving their products and my physiotherapy team have ordered a device which will help me to walk further and rest as necessary along the way.

In addition, I will continue my research into the latest scientific evidence about the healing power of personal and professional carers, the nature of emotions and their vital role in decision making, the brain's role in the creation and relief of pain, the restorative power of sleep and relaxation and the many ways in which we can change our lives for the better by altering our expectations, rewiring our brains' neural networks and controlling our feelings. Dr. Monty Lymon has just published a book entitled, *The Immune Brain* (2024) which I am looking forward to reading which explores a more holistic way of understanding what it means to be human. Such research enriches my life immensely.

In 2022 I felt that the vascular team of consultants were giving me a choice between having my left leg amputated or risk the probability of death. In 2023 I felt that Mrs. Rachel Sam was asking my permission to have my right leg amputated in a planned manner to have a better quality of life. Whatever the interpretations of the choices, I am glad I chose to have both my legs amputated and to be able to live the life I'm living. Today, I am focused on the question of how I can continue to improve the quality of my limbless life and serve others along the way.

ACKNOWLEDGMENTS

Without the care and support of my wife, Maureen this book would not have been able to be written. Her textual recommendations were also invaluable.

The many treatments provided by my daughter Larissa were invaluable in healing my muscles and providing various forms of relaxation and the cheerful companionship of my grandson Amir was inspiring to say the least.

The influence of Dr. William E. Hall my psychological mentor and role model is present in all the material devoted to the healing power of good relationships.

The work of Dr. Michael Mosley, Professor Luke O'Neil and Professor Russell Foster were a rich source of data relating to our circadian rhythm and, sound sleep and the former two, on the medicinal power of laughter.

The work and research of Professor Lisa Feldman Barrett and Leonard Mlodinow were heavily relied upon, when it came to the nature of emotions and the latest neuroscience concerning the brain.

Many insights into the science of pain and the brain were provided by the research of Dr. Monty Lyman.

The experience of being cared for by such dedicated and

delicate professional experts over the last four and a half years deserve my deepest gratification and include the team of podiatrists from Solihull, Balsall Common and Shirley, particularly Mark Poyner and Sandeep; the Senior Vascular Consultant, Mrs. Rachel Sam and the physiotherapy team at Selly Oak Rehabilitation Centre, Birmingham led by Dr. Ramamurthy and Liz Woods assisted by Emma, Hannah, Geoff, Mtumbi, Kat and Cloe.

Thank you all.

ABOUT THE AUTHOR

Jim Meehan is a retired Positive British Chartered Psychologist, Author and Poet. His fifty-year career was spread equally working in the United Kingdom in the Human Resources department of the Rover Car Manufacturing Company and in the United States working for Talent Plus an International Human Resources Consultancy, headquartered in Lincoln, Nebraska.

Although he was diagnosed as suffering from Type II diabetes in 1996 at the age of fifty-three he maintained a very active lifestyle. He was a keen mountain walker, an enthusiastic cyclist who rode 105 miles through Death Valley, California at the age of sixty-two and for his seventieth birthday ran the Chicago marathon.

However, his health took a turn for the worse when due to the complications of Type II diabetes, poor blood circulation and sepsis his left leg was amputated below the knee in March 2022 and his right leg was amputated below the knee in April 2023.

During his recovery he decided to publish this book about his health and fitness story, prior to and following his amputations in order to help others, both amputees and full-bodied adults alike, to benefit from his experience and coping strategies and enable them, to some extent, live a fuller, happier and healthier life.

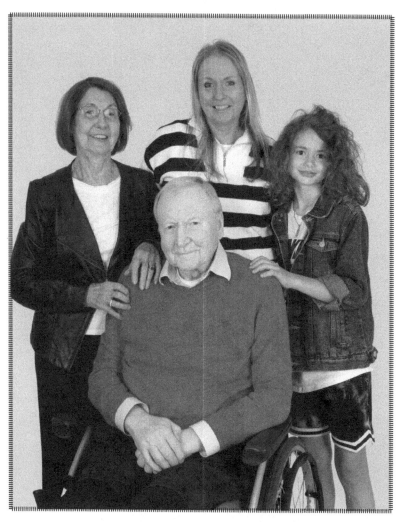

Photo 5. Family portrait. Left to right, Maureen, Jim, Larissa and Amir.

NOTES

Part One
My Health and Fitness Journey

1. **Enough is Enough** is one of the poems included in *Armless Hugs* by Jim Meehan published in 2020 and revised in 2023 by iUniverse, page 2.

Part Two
Step One
Embracing the healing power of good healing relationships

1. **Picture a World** is one of the poems included in *Armless Hugs* by Jim Meehan published in 2020 and revised in 2023 by iUniverse, page 55.
2. **"We have shaped an idea of a 'human being'** .... by Carlo Rovelli in *The Order of Time* published by Penguin Random House UK in 2019, pages 152-154.
3. **"We live longer if we have close, supportive relationships,"** ....by Lisa Feldman Barrett in *Seven and a Half Lessons About the Brain*, published by Picador UK in 2020, pages 85-88.

4. **"Every man is in certain respects"** .... by Clyde Kluckhohn and Henry A. Murray eds. *Personality in Nature* published by Knopf,1953: New York.

5. **"People who have friends"** .... by K.W. Choi et al. in The American Journal of Psychiatry, Vol.177, No 10. 2020.

6. **"They are also less likely to die"** .... by J. Holt-Lundstad et al. in PLOS Medicine, Vol.7 No.7 2010, A. Steptoe.

7. **"When people are low in social connection"** .... by Juliane Holt-Lundstad, PhD, professor of psychology and neuroscience at Brigham Young University.

8. **"Blood pressure reactivity"** .... by J. Holt-Lundstat et al. Annals of Behavioral Medicine, Vol.33, No.3, 2007.

9. **"A review of 38 studies"** .... by C. Pezirkiandis et al. in Frontiers in Psychology, Vol.14, 2023: R. Bliezner et al. Innovation in Aging, Vol.13 No.1 2019.

10. **"Interactions with acquaintances"** .... by Sandstrom in Personality and Social Psychology Bulletin, Vol.40, No.7,2014 & Journal of Experimental Social Psychology Vol.102, 2022.

11. **"We can benefit by blurring"** .... by Marissa G. Franco, PhD at University of Maryland and author of *Platonic* and also in NBER Working Paper No.20794, 2014.

12. **Dr Michael Mosley,** in Just One thing-Laughter, BBC Radio 4, Wednesday 8th November 2023.

13. **Professor Luke O'Neil,** in *Humanology- A scientist's Guide to Our Amazing Existence* by Gill Books, pages 126-137, 2018.

14. **Beyond Loving** is a poem included in *Armless Hugs* by Jim Meehan published by iUniverse in 2020 and revised in 2023.

Step Two
Understanding the brain's role in pain creation and pain relief

1. **The Painful Truth** by Dr. Monty Lyman published by Penguin Random House in 2021.
2. **Flow-The classic book on the achievement of happiness** by Mihaly Csikszentmihalyi published by Rider 2002.
3. **The Expectation Effect- How Your Mindset Can Transform Your Life** by Daid Dobson published by Cannongate Books Ltd, in 2022.

Step Three
Using the Restorative Power of Sound Sleep

1. **"It reminds me of a diagram"** .... by Professor Anil Seth in his book Being You-A new Science of Consciousness published in the UK by Faber &Faber Ltd., page 38, 2021.
2. **"You can think about energy efficiency like a budget"** .... by Lisa Feldman Barrett in Seven and a Half Lessons About the Brain ibid pages 5-8.
3. **"Most adults wake between"** .... by Professor Luke O'Neil ibid. pages167-171.
4. The American company **The Sleep Foundation** I found to be a reliable scientific resource concerning the science of sleep and related matters.

Step Four
Building hope and determination

1. Charles 'Rick' Snyder's main text on hope is *The Psychology of Hope: You Can Get Here from There* published by awesome books in 2003.

2. Lisa Feldman Barrett describes in her book *How Emotions Are Made-The Secret Life of the brain,* the many ways in which people can change their emotions and become 'architects of their own experience'. Published in the UK by Macmillan in 2017.

3. Leonard Mlodinow in his latest book *Emotional-The New Thinking About Feelings,* brings us up to date with the science of emotions and how to use them to benefit our well-being. Published in the UK by Allen Lane in 2022.

INDEX

A

Affect, often known as core
  affect, 86
Amputation, left leg, xiii, 16,103
Amputation, right leg, xiii,17,103
Antrim Coast Road, 7, 8
Armless Hugs Poems, 21, 32, 51

B

Barrett, Professor, Lisa Feldman
  35, 36,85, 110
Beecher, Dr. Henry, 60
Bevan, Aneurin, 5
Brain as predictive machine,
  57, 87
Bryan Hospital, Lincoln,
  Nebraska, 10
Butler, Daivid & Mosely,
  Lorimer, 89

C

Carlin, John, 20

Csikszentmihalyi, Mihaly, on
  Flow, 58
Corkhill, Betsan on Knitting, 90

D

Death Valley, California,
  10,11,12, 103
Diabetes Type II, 9, 18, 19, 97

E

Emperor Federick II
  Hohenstaufen's
  experiment, 32
Expectation effect, 58

F

Friendship as described by Dr.
  Hall, 44
Four Elements of Friendship,
  45, 46
Foster, Professor Russell on
  sleep, 75-79

R

Ravindran, Dr. Deepak, 89
Relationship Rules, silver, gold
    and platinum, 40
Recent research on the
    healing power of good
    relationships, 43, 44
Robson, Dave on the expectation
    effect, 61
Roeke, Theodore, the
    Waking, 69
Rovelli, Carlo, 33, 34

S

Sam, Mrs. Rachel, xiii, 15,
    98, 102,
Saint Elizabeth Hospital,
    Lincoln, Nebraska, 11
Seth, Professor, Anil, 69, 70, 71
Sleep Well...Live Better, 73
Snyder, Professor, Charles,
    'Rick,'85, 91
Steenkamp, Reeva, 20
SWALLOWS Walking Club, 13

T

Talent Plus, 9, 10, 11, 13, 14, 34

W

West midlands Rehabilitation
    Centre 16, 17, 101

AFTERWORD

Unfortunately, a regular monthly blood test on 3rd June 2024 indicated two major concerns that resulted in me being sent to the Accident & Emergency Department at South Warwickshire NHS Hospital for urgent tests on Friday 7th June.

The first concern was that I was bleeding internally at a rapid level and the second concern was that my serum prostate level was abnormally high and a possible sign of prostate cancer. Accordingly, I was given two blood transfusions over the weekend and on Monday had an endoscopy which involved a camera being inserted through my throat to film my upper colon and stomach. Fortunately, there was nothing amiss so the doctors arranged a full body CT scan to examine my lower abdomen. The CT scan was clear although it did show a slightly enlarged prostate and some minor calcification in the bladder walls.

On Friday afternoon I was discharged from hospital and asked to attend as an outpatient at both the gastroenterological and urological departments of Solihull Hospital for further ongoing scrutiny.

It was with great sadness that I learned during my stay in hospital that Dr. Michael Mosley, referred to earlier, died from natural causes after disappearing on a walk on the Greek Island of Symi on the 5th June 2024 at the age of sixty-seven. My condolences go to his surviving wife, who is also a medical doctor and his three surviving children. He will be greatly missed by all those who benefitted from his advice and support, including yours truly.

Printed in the United States
by Baker & Taylor Publisher Services